Beate Carrière PT, CIFK
512 S. Euclid No. 4
Pasadena CA 91101, USA

ISBN 3-540-61144-4 Springer-Verlag Berlin Heidelberg New York

Library of Congress Cataloging-in-Publication Data
Carriere, Beate, 1943 – The Swiss ball: theory, basic exercises and clinical application /
Beate Carriere, with a foreword by V. Jauden, with a contribution by Renate Tanzberger.
p. cm. Includes bibliographical references and index.
    ISBN 3-540-61144-4 (alk. paper). – ISBN 0-387-61144-4 (alk. paper)
1. Exercise therapy. 2. Physical therapy. 3. Balls (Sporting goods) I. Tanzberger, Renate.
II. Title. [DNLM: 1. Exercise therapy – methods. WB 541 C316s 1997] RM 725.C37 1998
615.8' 2–dc21 DNLM/DLC for Library of Congress

Springer-Verlag Berlin Heidelberg New York
a member of BertelsmannSpringer Science+Business Media GmbH

© Springer-Verlag Berlin Heidelberg 1998
    Printed in Germany

Production: PRO EDIT GmbH, Heidelberg
Typesetting (Data conversion): K+V Fotosatz GmbH, Beerfelden
Cover Design: Künkel + Lopka Werbeagentur, Ilvesheim

SPIN 10877174 22/3111-5 4 3 2 – Printed on acid-free paper

To my father from whom I inherited the gift of the pen

To my mother who gave me the gift of adventure

To Susanne Klein-Vogelbach, who taught me to observe and analyze movement

To all my friends who supported me faithfully with encouragement and understanding

Foreword

I have known Beate Carrière for several years and have always been impressed by her deep understanding of the whole field of physiotherapy. In our discussions her questions and comments have been inspiring and demonstrate that her knowledge is not only based on reading but rather on life-long clinical practice and experience. Thus, it is no wonder that her book is exceptional, presenting the physiology, the pathophysiology, and a technical description of recommended exercises and their clinical application – and not as general recommendations but with convincing examples. All three of the sections are written in clear, understandable language.

The author discusses the use of the Swiss ball; however, she did not limit herself to a technical description. Instead she set out to discover the underlying physiological mechanisms and has succeeded in showing how a knowledgable physiotherapist can contribute to the development of physiotherapy as a science.

Though based on the concept of S. Klein-Vogelbach, Beate Carrière has added so many of her own exercises, descriptions, and explanations that we are justified in speaking about the Carrière concept of using the Swiss ball. What I appreciate in particular is her critical view and attempt to see the patient and his problems from all possible aspects. Therefore, she does not consider the Swiss ball program the one and only means of treatment but incorporates other approaches as well. Her knowledge of the various techniques commands respect, and her familiarity with both the American and European (mainly German) traditions makes this book attractive to readers from all parts of the world.

It was a real pleasure for me to read Beate's book and I am confident that others will feel the same.

Prague, September 1997 Professor Vladimir Janda
Director, Dept. of Rehabilitation Medicine
Charles University Hospital, Prague, Czech Republic

Preface

For many years I have been asked by students and physical therapy friends to write a book about the Swiss ball, my daily companion in treating patients. The Swiss ball has become a tool that I use to motivate patients, to make exercising easier for them and for the physical therapists, and to relieve the strain on *my own* back when I have a hard day at work.

The more that I taught and lectured about the Swiss ball, the more I wanted to understand *why* and *how* this tool can be used not only by the very ill and recovering patient but also by healthy individuals. I began to read up on the matter and realized increasingly how the ball helps to motivate and challenge patients, probably activating the limbic system as well as other systems in the brain.

During the course of my career I have encountered many treatment protocols which are utterly boring, and which provide little or no feedback or motivation to the patient. Proper use of the Swiss ball can help to solve these problems. Many patients are able to use the Swiss ball at home, enjoy the exercises, feel challenged, and receive instant feedback. This is very important at a time when efficiency of treatment and self-motivation as well as cooperation of the patient and family is required in order to achieve progress. Long hospital stays are rare, and paid physical therapy treatments are often limited to a few sessions. When a patient exercises at home, the therapist gains valuable time to perform other treatments which may help the patient to recover more quickly.

Although the Swiss ball is rarely used exclusively, and sometimes only for certain aspects of the treatment with very ill and recovering patients, it is also a great tool for healthy individuals who wish to stretch, mobilize, and move the body after sitting all day at work, and for persons who must stand or move in a posture which is less than ideal.

The book is organized in two parts. The first part provides the background – the "why" and "how" of using the Swiss ball; the second part provides clinical applications and patient examples. A glossary is provided at the end, defining most of the principal terms used through the text.

It is my hope that this volume will not only provide therapists, teachers, and students with ideas and inspire them to invent exercises which are safe and challenging for their patients, but also help patients and family to have fun, and the therapists to work more efficiently with them.

I am particularly grateful to Dr. Susanne Klein-Vogelbach, who was my mentor and teacher for many years. This book is based on her teaching of functional kinetics as it is taught in Europe.

I also thank Renate Tanzberger, a physical therapist from Munich, who contributed the chapter on pelvic floor exercises. I know no other person who has such a sensitive and profound understanding of this subject. Her concept of pelvic floor exercises is widely taught in Germany. Mrs. Tanzberger contributes exercises which are not known in the United States but have helped many patients with urinary incontinence.

My thanks are also extended to the many persons who have encouraged and supported me to write this book in English, which is not my mother tongue (an additional challenge). It would be impossible to name all my friends and colleagues who have lent me support.

My specific thanks go to the following: Mary Sheh, who 12 years ago composed the first manuscript from lectures that I presented; she also contributed most of the drawings here. Susanne Greengard, who served as a model and as a friend. All the patients and families who allowed me to take "real" patient pictures. Prof. Darcy Umphred, with whom I have had many personal discussions, and who was always ready to answer my many questions. Thanks for helping me to make this a better book! Prof. Dee Lilly Masuda, who reviewed a chapter and provided me with advice. Jennifer Ault and Margret Goetz who faithfully proofread and corrected what I put on paper. Naomi Shwarzer, the director of the Physical Therapy Department at Kaiser Permanente Hospital, who encouraged me and allowed me to adjust my schedule so that I could write, work, and teach. The staff of the Kaiser Permanente library, who helped me in the search for articles. Marga Botsch and Dr. T. Barton from Springer-Verlag in Heidelberg, for making the trans-Atlantic communication an easy task. Karin Hofheinz a dear friend and colleague who is now translating the text into German. (Note: In the text I refer to the therapist as "she" and the patient as "he" unless otherwise noted.)

Pasadena, October 1997   *Beate Carrière*

Contents

Glossary

Actio	Initial or primary movement impulse in an exercise that leads to the goal of the exercise
Activated passive buttressing	Limitation of a continuing movement by a countermovement (of a body weight such as an arm or leg) which is adjusted in its length by muscular activity
Active buttressing	Limitation of a continuing movement by a muscular (antagonistic) counteractivity
Axes of movement	The intersection at which two planes meet. In functional kinetics described as fronto-sagittal, fronto-transverse, sagitto-transverse planes
Base of support	Contact points of the body with the ball and/or floor
Bisecting plane	An imaginary plane (as described by Klein-Vogelbach) which helps the observer to evaluate the distribution of body weights and the potential accelerating and braking weights. The plane is vertical and at a right angle to the direction of movement and passes through the center of gravity
Body distances	Distances between various points of the body which can be observed when moving during exercises. Observation of these points assists the therapist in identifying and correcting faulty movement sequences

Body segment	Functional-kinetics term for one of the five functional units of the body: head/neck, arms/shoulder girdle, thorax, lumbar spine/pelvis, and legs
Bridging activity	Functional-kinetics term for a muscular activity directed against gravity in a bridge-type position of the body (e.g., on hands and knees for abdominal muscles)
Caudal direction	Direction towards the feet
Centric weight bearing	Sitting on the top of and in the center of the ball
Changing-location exercise	An exercise in which the starting position differs from the end position (also known as nonstationary exercise)
Closed kinetic chain	Muscle activity which goes from distal to proximal and involves co-contraction of antagonistic muscles
Conditio	Instruction(s) given to the patient to help reach the goal of the exercise in a desired response
Constant-location exercise	An exercise in which the base of support changes not at all or only minimally from the start to the end of the exercise (also known as stationary exercise)
Continuing movement	A movement impulse that moves through the body. It can be observed because it moves in a predictable manner if there are no movement or strength limitations. Faulty movement patterns deviate from the expected direction and are uneconomical
Cranial direction	Direction towards the head
Critical point of observation	Points of contact with the environment or within the body which can be observed to identify and correct faulty movement sequences
Distal point of observation	The location for observing movements at a hinged joint which is far away from the fulcrum but still

	connected to the lever; this generally offers the best view
Dorsal direction	Direction towards the back
Dynamic balance	Balancing despite an external challenge
Dynamic stabilization	Stabilizing several joints or a body segment through muscular activity while maintaining balance or moving in space
Evasive movement	Undesired, uneconomical substitution for a movement or continuous movement. It is a compensatory mechanism usually due to lack of strength, mobility, or skill
Fixed spatial point	When observing movement, a point of the body that remains stable in space. *Absolute*: the partial point is "fixed" and does not move at all. *Relative*: the spatial point moves minimally in space
Free play	Functional-kinetics term for an extremity suspended from the body when muscular activity is directed from proximal to distal in an open kinetic chain
Frontal plane	In neutral standing, the plane that extends from side to side and cranial/caudal direction, dividing the body into front and back
Fulcrum	Point of observation in a hinged joint; the pivot point of movement
Hanging activity	An activity in which a body segment or part thereof is suspended from another part of the body or an external suspension
Kinesthetic awareness	Awareness of body parts in relation to each other. *Static*: knowing where the parts of the body are even without seeing them. *Dynamic*: awareness of change in position of two body parts in their relation to each other

Limitatio	A summary of what is achieved through the conditio(s) – a muscle activity or balance reaction
Midfrontal plane	In standing, the plane that is oriented vertically in space, with its frontal aspect passing through the crown of the head and center of the body
Movement tolerance	Availability of movement. The range of movement which may be necessary for the movement or position to be carried out
Nonstationary exercise	Exercise in which the location changes from the starting to the end position (also described as location-changing exercise)
Off-center weight bearing	Weight bearing that is not in the center, but rather off center, in front or at the side of the ball
Open kinetic chain	Muscle activity which goes from proximal to distal such as in a "free play" function. The muscles "on top" of the open chain are activated against gravity
Parking function	Functional-kinetics term for a resting position or starting position of an exercise with a low economical muscular activity which is required to maintain that position
PhysioRoll	A double ball in the shape of a peanut (manufactured by Ledraplastic, distributed in the United States by Ball Dynamics International, Denver, CO)
Planes of movement	*Sagittal*: in neutral standing, the plane extending in a forward/backward and cranial/caudal direction, dividing the body into two sides (left, right). *Frontal*: in neutral standing, the plane extending from side to side and cranial/caudal direction, dividing the body into front and back. *Transversal*: in neutral standing, the plane extending

	in a forward/backward and side to side direction, dividing the body into upper and lower parts
Plane of symmetry	In standing, a sagittal plane that passes through the crown of the head and the center of the body, dividing the body into two equal sides
Potential mobility	Functional-kinetics term to describe a constant readiness of muscles to react and adjust to movement changes
Pronation	Hand/forearm turned palm down
Prone position	Lying on the abdomen, face down
Reactio	The response to the initial movement impulse; an automatic balance reaction in response to the actio. The goal of the exercise lies in the reactio
Rostral direction	Direction towards the nose
Sagittal plane	In neutral standing, the plane that extends in a forward/backward and cranial/caudal direction, dividing the body into two sides (left, right)
Sit'n'Gym	A Swiss ball with rubber spikes to prevent rolling away (distributed in the United States by Ball Dynamics International, Denver, CO)
Sitfit	A flat ball that can be used as a cushion or for balance training (distributed in the United States by Sissel Orthopedic Products, Temecula, CA)
Splinting	Tightening of muscles to guard against movement; it can be caused by either fear or injury
Stabilizer	Plastic dish which can be placed under the ball to prevent it from rolling away when the patient loses contact with the ball (distributed in the United States by Sissel Orthopedic Products, Temecula, CA)

Static balance

Ability to balance without external challenge

Stationary exercise

Exercise in which the location changes not at all or only minimally over the base of support (also known as constant-location exercise)

Supination

Hand/forearm turned palm up

Supine position

Lying on the back, face up

Supporting function

Functional-kinetics term for a closed kinetic chain activity with a high economical muscular activity. Increased pressure can be felt under the part of the body which supports more than its own weight

Tentacle

Any part of the body that reaches out (in a "free play" function)

Transversal plane

In neutral standing, the plane that extends in a forward/backward and side to side direction, dividing the body into upper and lower parts

Ventral direction

Direction towards the abdomen

Weight bearing

Full: the entire weight of the body may be supported. *Partial*: only part of the body weight may be supported. *Reduced*: part of the weight of a body segment or part thereof is supported and does not have to be lifted

1 History of the Swiss Ball

1.1 Introduction

The ball has been used in physical therapy for neurodevelopmental treatment for about 40 years (Oetterly and Larsen 1996). I first became familiar with it during my training with Berta and Karel Bobath in 1967 in London and extended my experience with it while working in Switzerland from 1968 to 1970 and from 1976 to 1984 in a physical therapy practice in Munich, Germany. In the physical therapy practice I began using the smaller Pezzi ball. At first this was used with children to facilitate movements while they were on the table or kneeling or sitting on a mat on the floor. I then began using the Pezzi ball to treat adult patients with orthopedic and neurological dysfunctions and to teach ball exercise classes to physical therapists.

During my training with Dr. Susanne Klein-Vogelbach in 1982–1983 I learned more about the applications of the Pezzi ball. Klein-Vogelbach, herself a physical therapist, was the director of the Physical Therapy School in Basel, Switzerland, from 1955 until her retirement in 1974. She was awarded an honorary medical degree by the University of Basel for her analytic work in physical therapy. Klein-Vogelbach's concept of "functional kinetics" (Klein-Vogelbach 1990a) is based on observing, analyzing, and teaching human movement. She integrated the use of the ball in her classes of functional kinetics and then developed ball exercises which she analyzed and published (Klein-Vogelbach 1990b). In the United States the Pezzi ball was known as the "Swiss ball" (although the balls were made in Italy), probably so named by the first American physical therapists who learned ball exercises in Europe, where Klein-Vogelbach and her ball exercises were already known.

In 1983 I became an instructor in functional kinetics in Switzerland and returned to the United States in 1984. By this time the ball had become an indispensable tool to me, especially in rehabilitation and with orthopedic and neurological outpatients. In the United States, however, I found the balls unused, except for therapists treating children with cerebral palsy, and often hidden somewhere in the corner of the physical therapy department. I began using the Swiss ball in rehabilitation, but not without a great deal of resistance. Once I asked a stroke patient to sit on the ball, and he answered, "I graduated from Stanford, I am not sitting on a stupid ball." Only when I explained to him how this could improve his balance and gait did he agree to try the requested exercise.

My next application of the Swiss ball was in pediatric intensive care, where I easily convinced the physicians of the benefit of using the ball, even for babies with multiple problems such as infantile botulism (Carrière 1989; Carrière and Broski 1989). While the physicians were on rounds, I arranged to have one such baby recovering from flaccid paralysis to sit on the ball despite intubation, a feeding tube, and multiple monitors. The oxygen saturation and heart rate of the patient were good, and the baby remained content, while head control and equilibrium reactions were facilitated.

The colleagues became very interested in the Swiss ball approach. One colleague, Mary Sheh, transcribed her notes of my first lecture on the use of the Swiss ball, and this was the beginning of our cooperation in writing a detailed handout for exercise classes using the Swiss ball, based on the work of Klein-Vogelbach (1990b).

Using the handouts made in cooperation with Mary Sheh, I began teaching classes on Swiss ball to physical therapists in the United States both at the university and in weekend courses, and continued teaching in Germany. Several therapists are now teaching Swiss ball classes in the United States, and many have incorporated at least some aspects of the Swiss ball concept into their treatment of patients with neurological or orthopedic dysfunctions, especially those requiring spinal stabilization.

The changes in the health care system around the year 1993 resulted in reduced treatment sessions and required increased efficiency at work and greater participation of patients and family during the healing process. If exercises had to be performed regularly at home before the next treatment session, it was important to motivate and challenge the patient and to make the exercises fun and cost effective. The Swiss ball, now readily available, became the ideal tool for many home exercises.

1.2 History of Literature on the Swiss Ball

Until 1990 very little literature was available on the Swiss ball. Klein-Vogelbach's book was first published in 1981 in Germany and has been popular ever since. Although the English translation of this work has not yet appeared, the videotape of Klein-Vogelbach's Swiss ball exercises (Klein-Vogelbach 1990c) is now available in the United States.

Davies (1990) described applications of the Swiss ball for patients with hemiplegia, and Day (1991) has done so for practicing squatting. Hypes (1991) published a manual on the use of the ball with children. In 1993 several articles appeared in publications dealing with physical therapy. Carrière and Felix (1993) presented factors regarding the role of body proportions and provided examples of exercises with the Swiss Ball. Carrière (1993) described the use of the Swiss ball in the hospital, and Marcks (1993) the use of the PhysioRoll for the facilitation of motor skills. Posner-Mayer (1995) recently published a guide for home exercise programs using the Swiss ball, including a detailed history of it. Further suggestions for using the Swiss ball are provided by Umphred (1995) and Carrière (1996).

The Swiss ball has become an accepted therapeutic tool, not only in physical therapy departments but also among personal trainers and those seeking to promote a healthy life-style. Swiss balls are no longer a rarity but are readily available for anyone wishing to explore their many uses.

References

Carrière B (1989) Frühkindlicher Botulismus, eine seltene Krankheit? Krankengymnastik 41: 647–651

Carrière B (1993) Swiss ball exercises. PT Magazine Phys Ther 9:92–100

Carrière B (1996) Therapeutic exercises and self correction program. In: Flynn TW (ed) The thoracic spine and rib cage. Butterworth, Boston, pp 289–310

Carrière B, Broski (1989) Infant Botulism. Clin Manage Phys Ther 9(1):20-23

Carrière B, Felix L (1993) In consideration of proportions. PT Magazine Phys Ther 4:56–61

Davies PM (1990) Right in the middle. Springer, Berlin Heidelberg New York

Day L (1991) The squat. Clin Manage Phys Ther 11:81–82

Hypes B (1991) Facilitating development and sensorimotor function: treatment with the ball. PDP, Hugo

Klein-Vogelbach S (1990a) Functional kinetics. Springer, Berlin Heidelberg New York

Klein-Vogelbach S (1990b) Ballgymnastik zur Funktionellen Bewegungslehre, 3rd edn. Springer, Berlin Heidelberg New York

Klein-Vogelbach S (1990c) Functional kinetics: Swiss ball videotape. Springer, Berlin Heidelberg New York

Marcks LK (1993) Using the PhysioRoll for the facilitation of motor skills. Pediatr Phys Ther (Fall):154–155

Oetterly S, Larsen C (1996) Physiotherapy. Z Schweiz Physiotherapeutenverbandes 6:23–35

Posner-Mayer J (1995) Swiss ball applications for orthopedic and sports medicine. Ball Dynamics International, Denver

Umphred DA (ed) (1995) Neurological rehabilitation, 3rd edn. Mosby, St. Louis

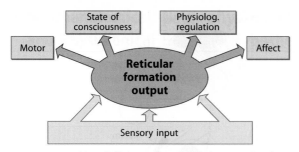

Fig. 2.2. Overview of the contribution of the reticular formation of the brain stem to various functional systems of the CNS. (From Schmidt-Thews (1995) Physiologie des Menschen, with kind permission from the publisher).

tem to voluntary muscles. Ascending and descending axons of the reticular formation have connecting collaterals and can therefore affect each other.

> There are at least four functions associated with the reticular formation (Fig. 2.2):
> 1. The ascending activating system of the reticular formation is the physiological basis for the levels of consciousness.
> 2. The reticular formation modulates segmental stretch reflexes and muscle tone.
> 3. The reticular formation is involved in the control of breathing and cardiac function.
> 4. Reticulospinal pathways modulate the sense of pain.

1. The ascending activating system of the reticular formation is the physiological basis for levels of consciousness.

> The ascending activating system of the reticular formation is connected to virtually all subcortical areas of brain, especially the thalamus (nucleus reticularis), an activating system which can influence the cortex.

The efferent neuronal connections of the reticular formation end at the spinal motoneurons and maintain their tonic activation during consciousness (Birbaumer and Schmidt 1995).

> The reticular formation modulates segmental stretch reflexes and muscle tone by means of the pontine and medullary reticulospinal tracts.

2. The pontine reticulospinal tract, when activated, enhances extensor muscle tone. This terminates near the motor nuclei of the ventral horn. The medullary reticulospinal tract inhibits extensor muscle tone when activated. This antagonistic activity is important for the control of motor function.

3. The reticular formation is involved in the control of breathing and cardiac function by sending axons of respiration-regulating neurons to the spinal cord where they control the activity of the motoneurons for muscles of respiration. In regulating the acceleration or depression of heart rate in response to an appropriate stimulus, neurons of the reticular formation are influenced by a variety of peripheral receptors and receive input from the hypothalamus and prefrontal cortex.

> The reticular formation therefore has a modulating effect on both the somatic motor and the autonomic motor system.

This integrative function provides adequate adjustment when the nervous system requires complementary support, for example, during exercises muscles metabolize at a higher rate in order to meet the nutritional demands. Heart rate and respiratory rate must increase or the striated muscle system would break down.

4. Reticulospinal pathways modulate the sense of pain. This is achieved by affecting the flow of information through the dorsal horn of the spinal cord (Role and Kelly 1991).

> Awareness of the complicated interactions of the reticular formation may help the therapist in treating patients. For example, a gentle rocking motion on a Swiss ball (resembling that of a rocking chair) can relax a person, while more vigorous bouncing or rocking may increase alertness (probably connecting the vestibular function with the reticular formation and a state of excitation).
>
> The bright color of the Swiss balls and the speed of movement may be further stimuli to the reticular formation and the limbic system, causing arousal.

> **EXAMPLES**
>
> A woman treated in our physical therapy department was originally very lethargic and difficult to arouse, but she started to respond when a Swiss ball was placed in her hands. She began throwing the ball to the therapist and became attentive and cooperative.
>
> A similar reaction was shown when a bright Swiss ball was placed near the foot of a lethargic patient in intensive care: the patient started kicking the ball and "woke up."

> A 45-cm Swiss ball was used to manage high muscle tone and increase the range of motion of the lower extremities of an 11-year-old boy (Fig. 2.3) who was comatose (Glascow Coma Scale 4–5; Jennett and Teasdale 1981). With the comatose child sitting at the edge of the bed, the Swiss ball supported the patient's arm while upright posture of the trunk and head was stimulated.

This is in accordance with Chusid (1985), who describes the reticular activating system (reticular formation) as being essential for arousal from sleep, wakefulness, alertness and focusing of attention, perceptual association, and direct introspection. Familiarity with the task, procedural programming, and arousal are all interrelated.

2.2 Cerebellum

Because of the cerebellum's close connection to the reticular formation, it is important to be aware of the functions of the cerebellum that correct and coordinate movements. The cerebellum receives impulses from the spinal cord, vestibular impulses from the inner ear, and impulses relayed by the vestibular nuclei. Proprioception and touch enter the cerebellum via the restiform body. Impulses from the cerebral cortex reach the cerebrocerebellum via the pontocerebellar pathways. The output is conveyed by the dentate nucleus of the cerebellum and from the cerebellum to the motor and premotor cortices. The cerebrocerebellum therefore plays a special role in the planning and initiation of movements.

> The cerebellum helps with postural and dynamic control due to its comparator function between what the brain wants, what the spinal generators send, and what the peripheral system experiences (Umphred personal communication).

Lesions to the cerebellum affect limbs and trunk on the ipsilateral side (Ghez 1991).

Silbernagl and Despopoulos (1983) use the example of a tennis player to demonstrate the integration and coordination ability of the cerebellum with the CNS, basal ganglia, and sensory pathways. When a tennis player serves, his body moves in the direction of the ball, which requires motor control, learned motor programs, and somatosensory feedback. The coordinated movement is then based on anticipatory feedforward programming which links multiple centers with the CNS and changes the program if feedback suggests that this is necessary. Equilibrium and acceleration information reaches the oldest part of the cerebellum, the archicerebellum (vestibulocerebellum), via vestibular nuclei. The vestibulocerebellum keeps the tennis

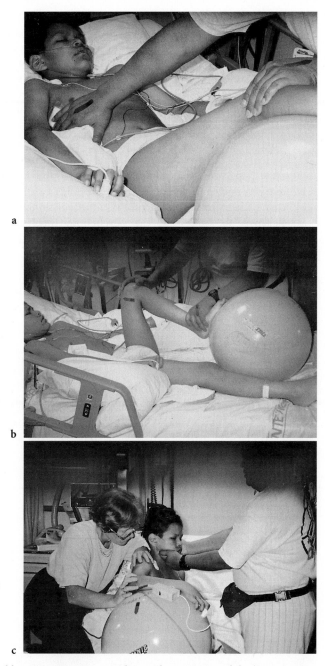

Fig. 2.3 a–c. An 11-year-old comatose patient. **a.** Side-to-side movement of the lower extremities can decrease muscle tone. **b.** Flexion and extension movement with proprioceptive stimulation to the left hip and knee joint to decrease extensor tone. **c.** Sitting a comatose patient up may affect respiration, heart rate, and alertness.

player oriented in space while he is balancing on one leg. Visual tracking analyzes the movement of the ball and assists in programming the motor responses of hitting the ball. The human vestibulocerebellum governs eye movement and body equilibrium during stance and during gait (Ghez 1991). The phylogenetically younger neocerebellum (cerebrocerebellum) processes incoming movement patterns from the cortex via the pons. It acts as a brake on volitional movements and skillfully coordinates intentional movements.

Control of voluntary movement can be lost not only by neurological patients but also by orthopedic patients and untrained persons. Visual cues (e.g., dots placed on the part of the body which should be moved) and auditory cues (e.g., clapping) can help accelerate the process of learning or relearning skillful volitional movements (Fig. 2.4). Because an injury to the cerebellum affects both automatic and learned movements, the patient may have difficulty with precision, coordination of movement, and equilibrium.

The Swiss ball may be an ideal tool in helping to restore these lost functions of movement and equilibrium.

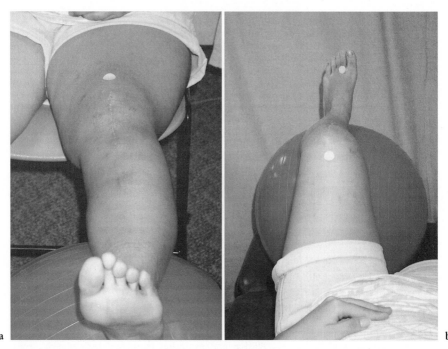

a   b

Fig. 2.4 a, b. Patient after knee surgery. **a.** Placing dots helps to visualize alignment of knee and foot. **b.** Bending the knee in good alignment is easier if dots are placed on foot and knee.

2.3 Vestibular System

Posture and balance are closely connected through the vestibular system of the brain and the inner ear. Two principal organs of equilibrium housed in the inner ear provide dominant afferent input to the vestibulocerebellum (Kelly 1991): (a) the semicircular canals and (b) the otolith organs. The semicircular canals signal changes in head position (Ghez 1991). Their arrangement in three-dimensional space allows detection of angular acceleration of the head in any of the three directions (Kelly 1991). The otolith organs detect linear accelerations and signal the position of the head with respect to gravity.

> Hair cells in the vestibular apparatus of the ear react to mechanical displacement induced by movement of fluid in the semicircular canals and the otolith organs. They translate the mechanical impulses into neural signs (Kelly 1991).

The vestibular portion of the eighth cranial nerve (vestibulocochlear) then relays the information from the semicircular canals and the otolith organs to the vestibular nuclei in the brain stem.

2.3.1 Vestibular Nuclei

The lateral vestibular (Deiters') nucleus receives input from the ear at its ventral portion while its dorsal portion receives input from the cerebellum and the spinal cord (Kelly 1991). Many of the cells of the dorsal portion of Deiters' nucleus send axons into the vestibulospinal tracts, which have a facilitatory effect on both γ- and α-motor neurons that innervate the limbs (extension of the legs and flexion of the upper extremities).

> Injury to the Deiters' nucleus can therefore result in decreased extensor tone.

The medial and superior vestibular nuclei also receive input from the inner ear. Neck movements are affected by the vestibulospinal tract, which participates in its reflex control.

Since neck and head movement must be correlated with eye movements, the medial and superior nuclei also participate in vestibulo-oculomotor reflex. Damage to hair cells in the semicircular canals has an effect on the vestibulo-oculomotor reflex: the patient becomes unable to keep a visual image fixed on the retina while moving the head (Goldberg and Eggers 1991).

The inferior vestibular nucleus also receives fibers from the inner ear and the cerebellum. Vestibulospinal and vestibuloreticular pathways add to the connections that together maintain posture and balance.

> The vestibular apparatus of the inner ear provides the vestibulocere-
> bellum and the vestibular nuclei with necessary information about
> the body's position and movement in space (Dewald 1987). Visual in-
> put is an alternate source of information about spatial relationships
> and can compensate for deficits associated with vestibular lesions.

All of these systems may be affected in patients with balance and postural
problems. The Swiss ball can be used to retrain some of these lost functions
by working on balance/equilibrium, muscle tone, and visual-spatial coordination. It must be remembered that although the vestibular system may be affected in balance, this is the least important; it is the somatosensory system
which is critical because it must match the environment with the stimulus.

2.3.2 Visual and Auditory Tracts

> Visual information is used whenever possible to guide and refine
> movement.

When all sensory systems are available, we tend to trust visual information
most and rely upon it for cognitive decisions, while using primarily the somatosensory input for feedforward procedural activities. Visual information
helps to refine a movement and complete a task (Magill 1989). The sensory
receptors of the eye transmit the information to the CNS.

> Actually *seeing* the object visually activates a motor program; vision
> is thus very involved in anticipatory behavior (Keele 1968).

Pursuing visually directed action means the continuous transformation of incoming visual stimuli into motor commands; not only does a target provide
information, but the absence of information about a target also has an effect
on the errors that are made (Jeannerod 1986).

> The ability of the head, eyes, and hand to move together provides a
> synergistic advantage which is missing when there is no head move-
> ment. Error is increased when the object is beyond the limit of the
> orbit of the eye (Jeannerod 1986).

Auditory input can prove very important, especially when a patient has visual-spatial deficits, which often result from lesions in the right hemisphere.
Patients with a right hemisphere lesion have increased movement latency

secondary to difficulty in determining the position of the target in extrapersonal space; these patients are also slightly slower than controls in initiating movement which began with an auditory stimulus (Goodale 1988; Goodale et al. 1990). All sensory information assists with establishing a consensus; therefore auditory cues can improve gait in patients with a hemiparesis (Brown et al. 1993).

All of the information above is important for physical therapists carrying out exercises with patients. The ability to move the head may improve the quality of the exercise. If the patient cannot move the head freely, it is important to position him so that he can see the target. A patient's leg can be placed on a Swiss ball to make it more visible.

> Dots can be put on the knee and foot to enhance this visual stimulus and make the patient more aware of the "target." Auditory cues can then be added to enhance the exercises. Later the patient should be able to perform the movement correctly without visual or auditory cues.

In patients with head injuries it is important to check the quality of voluntary movements to determine the extent of the lesion. Movement on the ipsilateral side, for example, is frequently affected in patients with a hemiplegia. Ipsilateral deficits are more common after left than after right hemispheric damage (Haaland et al. 1987).

A patient in supine position with a Swiss ball under the calf of the unaffected leg can be asked to move it in flexion and extension in a straight line at gait speed. This helps to detect problems of coordination and motor planning as well as potential changes in muscle tonus.

> Because the activity is contrived, it does not necessarily have a good carryover into other movements unless a functional activity follows.

2.4 Hypothalamus

The hypothalamus is the *master controller of the autonomic nervous system* (ANS; Loewy 1991; Goldberg 1988). Lesions in the hypothalamus can cause abnormal behavior, such as overeating or fear and rage reactions of the flight or fight response, which exhibits itself as motor behavior.

> The hypothalamus is also the primary regulator of endocrine functions and controls and balances homeostatic mechanisms.

It provides reciprocal interactions with most centers of the cerebral cortex, amygdala, hippocampus, pituitary gland, brain stem, and spinal cord. The subcortical limbic structures surround the hypothalamus and are vitally linked with each other and the hypothalamus (Umphred 1995). Autonomic reactions and maintenance of consciousness also involve the hypothalamus.

2.5 Thalamus

The hypothalamus and the thalamus together are referred to as the diencephalon, which is the part of the brain lying between the midbrain and the cerebral hemispheres. In the very complicated network of the brain the thalamus serves as *a sensory relay* and integrative center for many areas including the cerebral cortex, basal ganglia, hypothalamus, and brain stem.

> The diencephalon has a central role in sensation and motor control (Kelly et al. 1991).

Specific nuclei receive input about somatic sensation, audition, and vision. Motor functions are mediated and transmitted in the thalamus from the cerebellum and basal ganglia to the motor regions of the cortex.

2.6 Basal Ganglia

The basal ganglia are at the base of the cerebral cortex and include the caudate nucleus and putamen (together named corpus striatum), globus pallidus, substantia nigra, and subthalamic nucleus (Fig. 2.5). The basal ganglia affect motor circuits through their myriad miniloops to help specify the combinations, sequence, and direction of movements (Chevalier and Deniau 1990).

> The corpus striatum serves as the main entrance to this subcortical system, funneling information from the cortex, thalamic nuclei, and limbic system into the globus pallidus and the substantia nigra. The corpus striatum promotes arousal of the motor system and accounts for readiness in premotor networks (Chevalier and Deniau 1990).

The basal ganglia deal with a wider range of functions than the cerebellum (Brooks 1986).

> Purposeful movements are "planned" in the basal ganglia, which also adjust complex, simple, and semiautomatic functions.

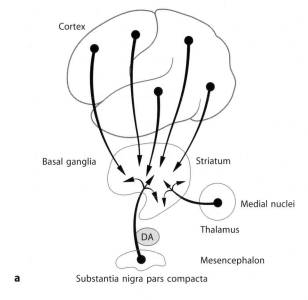

a

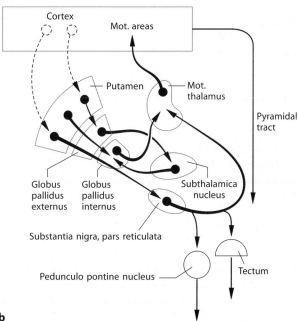

b

Fig. 2.5 a, b. Input and output pathways of the basal ganglia. The input to the basal ganglia is dominated by the cortex. In addition, the striatum is influenced by the substantia nigra, pars compacta (*SNc*), and the hypothalamus. The main output of the basal ganglia projects to the motor areas of the cortex through the motor nuclei of the thalamus. Only a small fraction of neurons exit directly to the spinal cord through the pendiculopontine nucleus and through the nuclei in the tectum. (From Schmidt-Thews (1995) Physiologie des Menschen, with kind permission of the publisher).

The caudate, for example, coordinates the overall motor plan. When this is destroyed, the ability to coordinate simultaneous or sequential motor acts is affected. The putamen, on the other hand, provides a link with the sensori-motor cortex and deals with scaling, adjusting, and updating programmed actions. The lack of support of the substantia nigra causes problems in patients with Parkinson's disease.

> There are many pathways, loops or circuits interlinking the neuron network, connecting and reconnecting the limbic and nonlimbic systems, and it is important to remember that all systems have several functions.

2.7 Autonomic Nervous System

Autonomic control consists of a reciprocal network between cell groups of the hypothalamus, basal ganglia, forebrain, and cerebral cortex, with the exception of the motor cortex, which does not participate in regulating the ANS (Loewy 1991).

> These centers control neuroendocrine and autonomic functions and innervate vagal and sympathetic preganglionic neurons.

This visceral and largely involuntary system can be differentiated into three divisions (Dodd and Role 1991):
– The sympathetic (thoracolumbar) division
– The parasympathetic (craniosacral) division
– The enteric division

The *enteric* division innervates the gastrointestinal tract, pancreas, and gall bladder. It plays a major role in homeostasis since it controls fluid transport, gastrointestinal blood vessel tone, motility, and gastric secretions.

> The *parasympathetic* division regulates primarily the internal environment, maintaining the basal heart rate, respiration, and metabolism under normal conditions. The *sympathetic* system reacts to external conditions by increasing the cardiac output, changing the body temperature and blood glucose and pupillary dilatation.

Both the parasympathetic and the sympathetic system innervate the enteric division.

Preganglionic neurons within the brain stem nuclei and the spinal cord activate postganglionic motor neurons located outside the CNS. Parasympathetic preganglionic neurons are located in the brain stem (cranial nerves III, VII, IX, X) and sacral segments (S2–S4).

Axons of the preganglionic cells of the sympathetic division exit the spinal cord from the first thoracic segment to the lower lumbar segments and connect to the paravertebral chain ganglia. Each preganglionic fiber synapses with many postganglionic fibers, ensuring that activation and coordination of several sympathetic neurons is possible at the same time.

> The close proximity of the paravertebral chain ganglia may be important for physical therapists. The technique called the "sympathetic slump" can load the sympathetic trunk (Slater et al. 1993, 1994). In the test for loading of the sympathetic trunk the subject is placed in a long sitting slump, the thoracic spine laterally flexed and rotated, and the cervical spine rotated to the same side.
>
> Results of the study support the hypothesis that the sympathetic slump increases sympathetic nervous system function (Slater et al. 1993, 1994). The test may help the therapist to understand sympathetically maintained pain.
>
> If this hypothesis is correct, it may explain why patients using the Swiss ball often report feeling well and aching less when the spine is mobilized in a similar manner as the sympathetic slump.

Figure 2.6 b demonstrates the use of the Swiss ball to support the trunk in this modified version; the patient, who had sustained multiple internal injuries in a motor vehicle accident, is shown mobilizing his spine and soft tissue structures.

2.8 Limbic System

The limbic complex plays an important role in motor control and learning (Umphred 1995). The better that physical therapists understand the complexity of the limbic system, the better they can adapt their treatment approach to the patient's needs.

> All major CNS systems interlock with and are codependent upon the environment (Umphred 1995; Fig. 2.7).

The limbic system, which consists of older structures surrounding the brain stem and branching out through their newer cortical connections, is vitally linked to the midbrain. The limbic system deals with biological drives such as feeding, drinking, and reproduction. Maternal and social behavior (including fight and flight decisions) are also attributed to the limbic system.

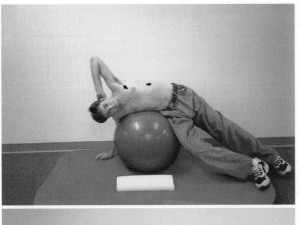

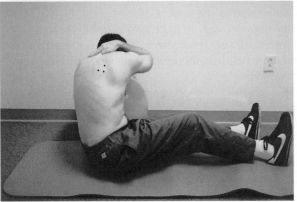

Fig. 2.6 a, b. Patient after MVA and internal injuries. **a.** Mobilizing spine and soft tissue. **b.** Modified sympathetic slump.

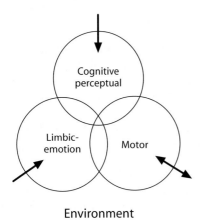

Fig. 2.7. Interlocking and codependency of major CNS systems with the environment. (From Umphred 1995, neurological rehabilitation, with kind permission from the publisher).

> The limbic system involves species-specific behavior and resulting emotional needs (Brooks 1986). It regulates the internal environment and thus life- and species-preserving activities and is important for the control of homeostasis.

Motivation has a great influence even over life-preserving activities. If motivated to do so, a person can find pleasure in overeating or starving.

> The limbic complex also allows one to select that which is to be remembered intellectually from past experience, which is very important for learning (Umphred 1995).

Umphred (1995) uses the mnemonic M^2OVE (adapted from Moore 1995) to label the functions of the motivational and memory part of the limbic system:

- M^2: *memory and motivation*, the drive to want to learn or to pay attention. A person who is permitted to attend some wonderful event is highly motivated to remember the time and date and to exert any necessary effort in order to attend it.
- O: *olfaction*, the sense of smell. In German the colloquial expression "I can't smell him" means that "I can't stand him." This definitely involves olfaction, which affects the limbic system directly. It is common knowledge that people are motivated and attracted by pleasant scents, and this fact is used by many industries.
- V: *visceral drives* such as thirst, hunger, and endocrine functions. A patient who fears a treatment may sweat profusely or feel faint, be unable to eat, etc.
- E: *emotions* relate to self-esteem, attitude, and social behavior. A patient may cry over a small scar or cry when asked to walk for the first time because he has difficulty emotionally in accepting the injury.

Because therapy succeeds best when the patient is motivated, it is always important to determine what would make the patient want to perform a task. The Swiss ball is a valuable tool in this respect. Almost everyone can be presumed to have played with a ball during childhood or even as an adult. This memory, along with the Swiss ball's bright color, texture, and shape makes it a valuable tool for inducing reaction/movement.

The patient may also be motivated by the fact that the Swiss ball facilitates movements by supporting part of the body weight. When used to challenge the patient, the ball can become a self-motivating tool. In Fig. 2.8a a patient is moving the operated right leg with the help of the ball 7 days after anterior cruciate ligament reconstruction; Fig. 2.8b shows the same patient 6 weeks after the surgery, finding the exercise "Cocktail Party" challenging.

A thorough description of the emotional circuitry of the amygdala as part of the limbic system is provided by Umphred (1995), who uses the abbreviation F^2ARV for a continuum of behavior:

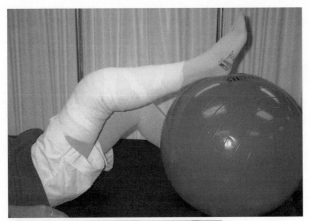

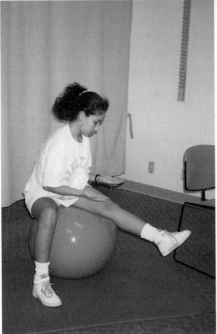

Fig. 2.8 a. A patient moves the right leg (which was operated) with the help of the left leg and the ball, 7 days after anterior cruciate ligament reconstruction. **b.** Six weeks after surgery the patient finds the exercise "Cocktail Party" challenging.

- F²: *fear/frustration*
- A: *anger*
- R: *rage*
- V: *violence*

Therapists are well aware of how important it is to deal properly with patients' emotions. Patients who feel safe can relax and participate in learning without strong emotional reactions (Umphred 1995).

Patients show greater willingness to learn, perform, and remember when they trust the therapist and feel safe. On the other hand, a patient can become very frustrated if the therapist is too forceful or too demanding. It may also be very difficult to motivate a patient who is mourning, depressed, or lacking in self-confidence.

Whether the patient is rigid or relaxed depends largely on his emotional state and on the interaction with the therapist. Exercising with the Swiss ball, however, can be a source of such fun that it becomes a motivating factor for almost any patient.

The amygdala and hippocampus are limbic structures involved in the memory aspect of learning (Kelly and Dodd 1991).

The amygdala deals with the emotional aspect (which differs from the motor memory) and the hippocampus with storage of memory. The amygdala and hippocampus have reciprocal connections as well as many other links to various vital centers of the brain. Degenerative changes in the hippocampus occur in patients with Alzheimer's disease and affect recent memory. The amygdala and other areas of the limbic system can also be affected by Alzheimer's pathology, causing dysfunctions such as uncontrollable appetite and violence (Goldman and Côté 1991).

Inattention, slowness, perseveration, impulsiveness, lack of inhibition, and lack of motivation are characteristic symptoms in neurological patients when the limbic system is affected.

These symptoms must be considered by the therapist when treating patients.

Neurochemical regulation of the limbic system takes place in its physiological center, the hypothalamus. The hypothalamus regulates body temperature, heart rate, blood pressure, and food and water intake. Lesions in the medial hypothalamus can cause huge weight gains and hostility, while lesions in the lateral hypothalamus lead to aphagia, hypoarousal, decreased sensory awareness, and depression (Umphred 1995).

There is a hierarchy of command in the complicated CNS. The flow of information through the limbic and sensorimotor system depends on the nature of the task to be carried out, on the subject's emotions, and on previous experience (Brooks 1986). While the two systems influence one other, emotional factors can override the sensorimotor system by controlling neuroendocrine and autonomic functions (Fig. 2.9).

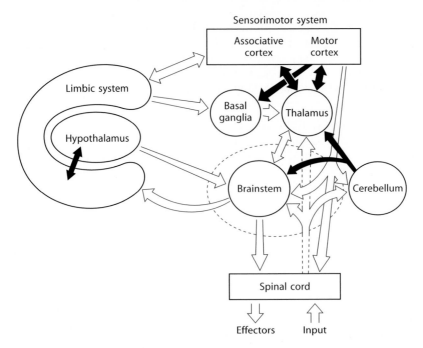

Fig. 2.9. Relationships between limbic and sensorimotor system. (From Umphred 1995, neurological rehabilitation, with kind permission from the publisher).

2.9 Sensorimotor System

The *association cortex* is the highest level of the sensorimotor command hierarchy (Brooks 1986). Although the motor system is today thought to work in terms of consensus, the crucial role of the associative cortex in motor regulation cannot be disputed. It is involved in the perception and conception of motor actions. It is here that strategies are developed and then conveyed to the prefrontal and parietal areas of the sensorimotor cortex which are in the middle level of the projection system. The association cortex of one side influences both sides of the periphery (Zilles and Rehkämper 1994). The premotor area assists in guiding the specifics of movement via the spinal cord to the entire musculoskeletal system – through the basal ganglia, cerebellum, and entire neocerebral cortex (which projects information to the basal ganglia; Brooks 1986). The parietal cortex (areas 5 and 7) integrates the three-dimensional sense and body image to assist in coordination of movement.

> All of these regions have reciprocal connections to one another and project to the primary motor cortex (area 4), which is the main source of descending fibers of the corticospinal tract and other fibers which project to the spinal cord, the pons, and other parts of the brain stem, thalamus, and basal ganglia (Zilles and Rehkämper 1994).

The motor cortex assists in modulating the spinal cord when implementing intended movements and posture. The "knowledge" of the overall purpose contained in the motor plan is not shared by all parts of the brain that carry it out (Brooks 1986).

> Preparatory messages (from areas 2 and 5 and some neurons in area 4) reach the spinal cord 0.1 second before the beginning of movement (Brooks 1986). It may therefore be important for the therapist to give patients some time to concentrate on the movement which is expected of them.

The afferent and efferent neurons (a- and γ-motor neurons to muscles of the trunk and limbs) and several interneurons are part of the basic soft wiring at the segmental level (Jewell 1995). The sum of all synaptic events determines whether the next neuron fires.

> The vestibular, proprioceptive, and visual systems play an important part in determining dynamic posture.

These systems provide information regarding the sense of "uprightness" or lack thereof. Swiss ball exercises such as the "Cowboy" (Sect. 9.1) and the "Scale" (9.2) stimulate the sensory systems and may also improve balance, although the balance is initially limited to the activity itself.

> Damage to the interneurons involved in producing posture can cause rigidity (Jewell 1995).

Approximately 75%–95% of the corticospinal fibers cross to the other side of the body at the level of the medulla, descending in the dorsolateral part of the white matter (Hummelsheim 1994). The remaining fibers cross at the spinal level and may also send ipsilateral collaterals. This might explain compensation for damaged fibers, thus improving function.

> Adults with damage to the corticospinal tracts usually lose fine motor control to the hand.

Spinal programs compete for available synaptic spots (Brooks 1986). The amount of transmitter fluid released from the synaptic endings increases with frequent use.

> The rule of "use it or lose it" applies to these spinal programs and perhaps for all neuronal systems. Even the simplest human movement can be improved through practice (Gottlieb et al. 1988).

Regular exercise is thus important in patients with CNS disorders (Hummelsheim and Neumann 1991).

Upon injury to the CNS, part of the mechanism of neural plasticity of the CNS is its ability to demask or activate silent, unused synapses (Mauritz 1994). After a lesion (e.g., stroke) axon collaterals sprout and bilateral tracts become activated.

> Motor learning increases the amount of cortical synapses and induces changes in the synaptic cortical connections, and it may therefore be significant in the rehabilitation of a patient (Asanuma and Keller 1991).

Sensory information is transmitted from the peripheral nervous system to the spinal cord and the brain via afferent neurons by tapping, touching, stroking, or giving hot or cold stimuli to the muscle, tendon, or skin (Fig. 2.10). Pain and pressure is perceived by cutaneous receptors and is also transmitted through afferent neurons. The muscle spindle, golgi tendon organ, and cutaneous receptors assist the spinal cord in assessing and calculating how much the agonist should contract and the antagonist should lengthen (Brooks 1986). The task and environment within determine which of the tasks are to be performed.

To simplify, the afferent pathways, which are in the white matter of the spinal cord, relay sensory information to the brain, while the descending pathways in the white matter of the spinal cord relay motor instructions from the brain (Goldberg 1988). The gray matter of the spinal cord contains many neuronal cell bodies and synapses. However, the earlier view of the spinal cord as resembling a telephone cable transmitting messages from the muscle to the brain is now rejected (Magill 1989).

> The spinal cord is part of a very complex system that interacts with a variety of systems and may itself be critically involved in the movement process.

Maintaining the mobility and flexibility of the spine is very important (Fig. 2.11). A key concept in understanding faulty movement patterns is that of *"relative flexibility/stiffness"* (Sahrman 1993). Movement following the

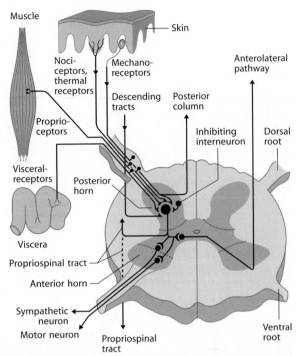

Fig. 2.10. Example of interconnection of the somatovisceral afferences in the spinal cord. Different types of afferences enter the posterior root and stimulate the neurons in the posterior horn. From there efferent fibers of the propriospinal tract are activated as well as afferent tracts (anterolateral pathways), and efferent sympathetic and motor neurons. Collaterals of the group I and II afferences ascend in the posterior column of the white matter directly to the medulla oblongata. The neuron in the posterior horn is inhibited by the descending tracts from the brain and inhibiting interneurons. (From Schmidt-Thews (1995) Physiologie des Menschen, with kind permission from the publisher).

path of least resistance is based on a law of physics. A patient with stiff segments in the spine moves where it is easy to move, and does not move where it is difficult to do so, causing strain to the already mobile segment.

Pathological problems of the nervous, muscular, or skeletal system can produce movement dysfunction with a variety of signs and symptoms.

> Faulty movement can also induce pathology and not be merely the result of pathology (Sahrman 1993).

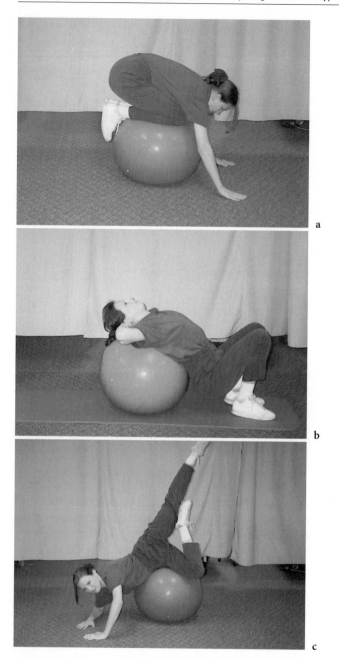

Fig. 2.11 a–c. A person with a healthy spine in extension, flexion, and rotation using a Swiss ball.

> Joint pain should not be considered as strictly a local problem but rather as a disorder that involves the motor system in general (Janda 1986, 1991). Special attention must be paid to muscles.

These are the effectors that respond to stimuli from the CNS and also react to changes of position in peripheral joints.

> Impaired central nervous system motor planning affects muscles and is an important precondition for chronic pain syndromes (Janda 1986, 1991).

Similarly, efferent tracts from the brain stem regulate incoming peripheral afferent input and thus the patient's perception of pain and its effect on the motor generators (Umphred personal communication).

The vertebral canal lies posterior to the center of motion of each vertebral segment (Inman et al. 1942). Because of its relationship, flexion of the spinal column leads to elongation while extension leads to shortening of the vertebral canal. When moving the spinal column from full flexion to full extension the total change in its length is approximately 7 cm.

> The dural sac surrounding the spinal cord undergoes the same extent of elongation, because it is firmly held at both of its extremities. The movement of the dura is directly transmitted to the spinal nerves (Inman et al. 1942).

Studies of vertebroradicular and vertebromedullar dynamics show that the vertebral canal lengthens by 9 cm during the transition from hyperextension to hyperflexion, with maximal mobility usually at C6 and L4 (Louis 1981). In hyperflexion the dural sac is stretched while in hyperextension it demonstrates transverse folds, notably in the interlaminar spaces. Maximal cord displacement relative to the walls of the vertebral canal are around C1 (7 mm caudally), T1 (7 mm cranially) and L1 (10 mm caudally).

Mobilization of the neural and surrounding tissues has received substantial attention by Australian therapists. Maitland (1986) describes the slump test as part of the evaluation of the spine. Butler and Gifford (1989) describe the concept of mechanical tension in the nervous system, and Butler (1991) devoted an entire book to mobilization of the nervous system.

> Due to the multilayered mesh of the nervous system in the body and its referral potential, no area of the body is exempt from symptoms arising from injury to the nervous system (Butler 1991). Therapists must be aware of symptoms which do not fit the pattern.

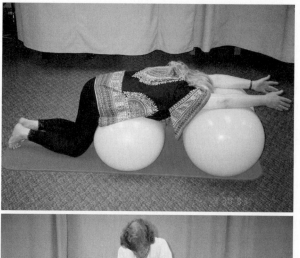

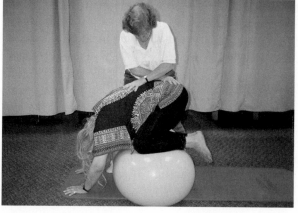

Fig. 2.12 a, b. A patient 6 months after low back surgery. **a.** Mobilizing the spine into extension over two PhysioRolls. **b.** Mobilizing the spine into flexion using one PhysioRoll.

EXAMPLES

For example, a patient 6 months after surgery to her low back complained of continuing back and leg pain until her spine was gently "mobilized" and the soft tissue moved into flexion, extension, lateral flexion, and rotation using the Swiss ball (Fig. 2.12).

There are many other physical therapy techniques and approaches to stimulate the sensory motor system. Rood (1954) recommendes brushing, cold applications, pressure, touch, vibration, and stretch. Klein-Vogelbach (1991) uses complex movement patterns stimulating joint, muscle, and tendon receptors. Bouncing with the Swiss ball triggers proprioceptive pathways of the CNS. The ball is also used for stretching and facilitation of movements and can be used for joint mobilization (see Chap. 8). Bobath (1978) prefers tapping, stroking, and reflex inhibition. Vojta (1981) stimulates afferents to obtain an efferent response during reflex locomotion. Brunkow's recommendation (Bold and Grossmann 1983) is automatization of normal movements and cocontractions of muscles of the extremities to facilitate stabilization of the trunk muscles, sometimes with stimulation of cutaneous mechanoreceptors. Proprioceptive neuromuscular facilitation (Adler et al. 1993) is based upon muscle stretch and compression and activation of muscle chains. Feldenkrais (1972) seeks to change faulty movement patterns by increasing awareness of movement.

> All approaches can provide input to the CNS and stimulate dormant or poorly used spinal programs. Motor and neighboring sensory neurons are sensitive to inputs from the periphery and can adapt in remarkable ways during training, contributing to spontaneous and training-induced recovery of function (Dobkin 1993).

2.10 Physiological Responses

The Swiss ball can be very beneficial in very ill patients. Those in intensive care can suffer from generalized weakness whether on the respirator, after abdominal surgery, with Guillain-Barré syndrome, after a stroke, with chronic obstructive pulmonary disease (COPD), or after organ transplants.

> Understanding how energy is transformed may help therapists to work more effectively with these patients and to stimulate the body's vital systems.

A detailed description of the way in which energy is transformed from one form into another, and how this is related to the performing of work is provided by McArdle et al. (1986) and Wasserman and Whipp (1975). In humans free energy produced during cell respiration is used for muscle contraction (mechanical), biosynthesis of cell molecules (chemical), and concentration of chemicals in intra- and extracellular fluids (transportation). Adenosine triphosphate is a special carrier of free energy.

A complicated mechanism of reactions, for example, the Krebs cycle, transforms food into energy to be used in chemical and biological work such as secretions from glands, digestion, muscle contraction, nerve transmission, circulation, and synthesis of new tissue.

The availability of oxygen is important during these chemical processes of energy metabolism since this determines the aerobic energy released during exercise. If oxygen delivery is inadequate during strenuous exercises, there is a temporary buildup of lactic acid as well as insufficient carbon dioxide clearance, which is produced from metabolism and buffering of lactic acid.

> If the level of lactic acid continues to increase in the muscle and the blood, the patient becomes fatigued and may have to stop or slow down until the oxygen demand is met.

Lactic acid can then be recycled into pyruvic acid, which again can be used as an energy source. Lactic acid levels in the blood of healthy persons performing light or moderate exercise remains fairly stable, although oxygen consumption may increase, and persons lacking regular exercise may take longer to reach a steady rate of oxygen consumption (steady rate of VO_2).

> With strenuous exercises more oxygen is needed in the recovery period not only to help the chemical processes but also:
> - To reload the blood as it returns from the muscles which were exercised
> - Because the respiratory muscles work harder and require more oxygen
> - Because the heart works harder and requires more oxygen
>
> Moderate exercise during the recovery period from strenuous exercise may help the removal of lactic acid.

Just as developing cardiovascular fitness is important for the conditioning of athletes (Latin 1990), some cardiovascular training may also benefit the patients in intensive care.

> When performing exercises with a very ill patient, it is important to remember that an exercise which involves only light or moderate effort from a healthy person may be strenuous for a patient.

It is necessary to monitor the respiratory rate, heart rate, and O_2 saturation and to observe the electrocardiogram. Most of our clients in intensive care have multiple problems affecting the cardiovascular and respiratory system directly or indirectly combined with metabolic and neuromuscular disorders and/or surgery.

The use of the ball to unload the muscles and thus provide a more moderate exercise environment has the potential of helping the muscles regain power and endurance without creating excessive chemical imbalance.

> Therapists should check the monitors frequently while the patients are performing exercises and recognize signs of distress or poor tolerance to the exercise, such as shortness of breath, fatigue, poor skin color, and increased perspiration. Lack of cardiovascular fitness may present symptoms resembling those of an underlying disease.

Nery et al. (1983) report that dyspnea is more prevalent in COPD patients during exercise due to a reduction in ventilatory capacity. Patients with mitral valve disease complain of general fatigue and pain in leg muscles when reaching their limit of exercise. Capacity is reduced secondary to the compromised cardiovascular performance. Physical therapists must also remember that arm exercises require greater O_2 consumption and result in a greater physiological strain.

Exercising is beneficial to COPD and asthmatic patients (Casaburi et al. 1991; Cochrane and Clark 1990; Cooper 1995). Casaburi et al. (1991) studied ventilatory response to exercise and found a strong relationship between training-induced decreases in blood lactate and ventilation.

> Cochrane and Clark (1990) report that exercises performed submaximally and with controlled intensity significantly improve fitness and cardiorespiratory performance in asthmatic patients.

Their study showed physiological improvements after training in maximal work capacity. Oxygen delivery throughout submaximal exercise was improved, resulting in a decrease of blood lactate and carbon dioxide output. The study also showed improvements in cardiorespiratory performance, including reduction in breathlessness.

Exercise training is very important in patients with COPD and offers the following benefits (Cooper 1995):
- Improved *aerobic capacity*
- Increased *muscle strength*
- Improved *ventilatory muscle strength*
- Improved *neuromuscular coordination*
- *Desensitization to dyspnea*

Cooper (1995) maintains that higher intensity exercise is likely to produce a greater physiological training effect, but that low intensity exercise also can be associated with significant physiological changes and with clinical improvement.

> Exercising with oxygen may improve exercise capacity and reduce dyspnea. Cooper recommends providing supplemental oxygen when O_2 saturation falls below 90%.

Bedridden, deconditioned patients in intensive care generally benefit from active exercises adjusted to their physical condition. For example, a Swiss ball placed under the leg enables the patient to move the leg actively without having to lift it (Fig. 2.13).

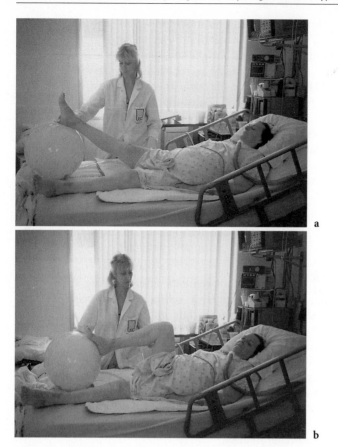

Fig. 2.13 a, b. Patient in intensive care post myocardial infarction and cerebral vascular accident actively moving nonparetic right leg in abduction and in flexion of the hip.

> This greatly reduces energy expenditure because the weight of the leg rests on the ball, reducing the body mass to be moved.

The patient can move one or both legs in different directions and at different speeds. The intensity can be varied, and resistance can be added as the patient improves.

2.10.1 Valsalva Maneuver

The Valsalva maneuver (straining and holding the breath while closing of the glottis) causes intrathoracic pressure to increase, compressing the veins in the thoracic region. This results in reduced venous return to the heart (McArdle et al. 1986). A sharp increase in blood pressure followed by a sudden drop is thought to be caused by the associated straining when an isometric type of exercise is performed. The patient may complain of dizziness or "spots before the eye" and may even faint with the Valsalva maneuver. This should be avoided in patients with cardiovascular problems and in those admitted for high-risk pregnancy. Again, the ball enables the patient to move without having to strain. Breathing exercises may be used to accompany the active Swiss ball movements.

References

Adler SS, Beckers D, Buck M (1993) PNF in practice. Springer, Berlin Heidelberg New York

Asanuma H, Keller A (1991) Neurobiological basis of motor learning and memory. Concepts Neurosci 2:1–30

Birbaumer N, Schmidt RF (1995) Wachen, Aufmerksamkeit und Schlafen. In: Schmidt RF, Thews G (eds) Physiologie des Menschen, 26th edn. Springer, Berlin Heidelberg New York, pp 141–153

Bobath B (1978) Evaluation and treatment, 2nd edn. Heinemann, London

Bold RM, Grossmann A (1983) Stemmführung nach R. Brunkow. Enke, Stuttgart

Brodal A (1981) Neurological anatomy. Oxford University Press, New York

Brooks VB (1986) The neural basis of motor control. Oxford University Press, New York

Brown SH, Thaut MH, Benjamin J, Cooke JD (1993) Effects of rhythmic auditory cueing on temporal sequencing of complex arm movements. Abstr Soc Neurosci 19:546

Butler DS (1991) Mobilisation of the nervous system. Churchill Livingston, New York

Butler DS, Gifford LS (1989) The concept of adverse mechanical tension in the nervous system. I. Testing for 'dural tension.' Physiotherapy 75:622–629

Casaburi R, Patessio A, Ioli F, Zanaboni C, Donner CF, Wasserman K (1991) Reductions in exercise lactic acidosis and ventilation as result of exercise training in patients with obstructive lung disease. Am Rev Respir Dis 143:9–18

Chevalier G, Deniau JM (1990) Disinhibition as a basic process in the expression of striatal functions. Trends Neurosci 13:277–280

Chusid JG (1985) Correlative neuroanatomy and functional neurology. Lange Medical, Los Altos

Cochrane LM Clark CJ (1990) Benefits and problems of a physical training programme for asthmatic patients. Thorax 45:345–351

Cooper CB (1995) Determining the role of exercise in patients with chronic pulmonary disease. Medicine and science in sports and exercise. Am Coll Sports Med, June:147–157

Dewald JPA (1987) Sensorimotor neurophysiology and the basis of neurofacilitation therapeutic techniques. In: Brandstater ME, Basmajian JV (eds) Stroke rehabilitation. William and Wilkins, pp 109–182

Dobkin BH (1993) Neuroplasticity – key to recovery after central nervous system injury. West J Med 159:56–60

Dodd J, Role LW (1991) The autonomic nervous system. In: Kandel ER, Schwartz JH, Jessell TM (eds) Principles of neural science, 3rd edn. Elsevier Science, Amsterdam, pp 761–775

Feldenkrais M (1972) Awareness through movement. Harper & Row, New York

Ghez C (1991) The cerebellum. In: Kandel ER, Schwartz JH, Jessell TM (eds) Principles of neural science, 3rd edn. Elsevier Science, Amsterdam, New York, pp 626–646

Goldberg ME, Eggers HM, Gouras P (1991) The ocular motor system. In: Kandel ER, Schwartz JH, Jessell TM (eds) Principles of neural science, 3rd edn. Elsevier Science, Amsterdam, New York, pp 660–678

Goldberg S (1988) Clinical neuroanatomy. MedMaster, Miami

Goldman J, Côté L (1991) Aging of the brain: dementia of the Alzheimer's type. In: Kandel ER, Schwartz JH, Jessell TM (eds) Principles of neural science, 3rd edn. Elsevier Science, Amsterdam, New York, pp 974–983

Goodale (1988) Hemispheric differences in motor control. Behav Brain Res 30:203–214

Goodale, Milner AD, Jakobson LS, Carey DP (1990) Kinematic analysis of limb movements in neuropsychological research. Can J Psychol 44(2):180–195

Gottlieb GL, Corcos DM, Jaric S, Agarwal GC (1988) Practice improves even the simplest movements. Exp Brain Res 73:436–440

Haaland KY, Harrington DL, Yeo R (1987) The effect of task complexity on motor performance in left and right CVA patients. Neuropsychologia 25 (5):783–794

Hummelsheim H (1994) Mechanismen der gestörten Motorik. In: Mauritz KH (ed) Rehabilitation nach Schlaganfall. Kohlhammer, Stuttgart, pp 64–86

Hummelsheim H, Neumann S (1991) Regelmässiges Training ist das A und O. Psycho 17(6):385/19–388/22

Inman VT, John B de CM, Saunders MB (1942) The clinico-anatomical aspects of the lumbosacral region. Radiology 38:669–678

Janda V (1986) Muscle weakness and inhibition (pseudoparesis) in back pain syndromes. In: Grieve GP (ed) Modern manual therapy of the vertebral column. Churchill Livingstone, New York, pp 197–201

Janda V (1991) Muscle spasm – a proposed procedure for differential diagnosis. J Manual Med 6:136–139

Jeannerod M (1986) Mechanisms of visuomotor coordination: a study in normal and brain-damaged subjects. Neuropsychologia 24(1):41–48

Jennett B, Teasdale G (1981) Management of head injuries. Davis, Philadelphia

Jewell MJ (1995) Overview of the structure and function of the central nervous system. In: Umphred DA (ed) Neurological rehabilitation, 3rd edn. Mosby, St. Louis, pp 66–80

Keele SW (1968) Movement control in skilled motor performance. Psychol Bull 70(6):387–403

Kelly JP (1991) The sense of balance. In: Kandel ER, Schwartz JH, Jessell TM (eds) Principles of neural science, 3rd edn. Elsevier Science, Amsterdam, New York, pp 500–511

Kelly JP, Dodd J (1991) Anatomical organization of the nervous system. In, Kandel ER, Schwartz JH, Jessell TM (eds) Principles of neural science, 3rd edn. Elsevier Science, Amsterdam, New York, pp 273–295

Klein-Vogelbach S (1991) Therapeutic exercises in functional kinetics. Springer, Berlin Heidelberg New York

Latin RW (1990) Preseasonal conditioning. In: Melhon MB, Walsh WM, Shelton GL (eds) The team physician's handbook, chap 6. Hanley and Belfus. Philadelphia, pp 27–33

Liebman M (1991) Neuroanatomy made easy and understandable. Aspen, Gaithersburg

Loewy AD (1991) forebrain nuclei involved in automatic control. In: Holstege G (ed) Role of the forebrain in sensation and behavior. Elsevier, Amsterdam, pp 253–268

Louis R (1981) Vertebroradicular and vertebromedullar dynamics. Anat Clin 3:1–11

Magill RA (1989) Motor learning: concepts and applications, 3rd edn. Brown, Dubuque

Maitland GD (1986) Vertebral manipulation, 5th edn. Butterworths, London

Mauritz KH (1994) Plastizität als Grundlage der Funktionswiederherstellung. In: Rehabilitation nach Schlaganfall. Kohlhammer, Stuttgart, pp 56–63

McArdle WD, Katch FI, Katch VL (1986) Exercise physiology. Lea & Febiger, Philadelphia

Moore JC (1995) Limbic complex. In: Umphred DA (ed) Neurological rehabilitation, 3rd edn. Mosby, St. Louis, pp 92–117

Nery LE, Wasserman K, French W, Oren A, Davis JA (1983) Contrasting cardiovascular and respiratory responses to exercises. Chest 3:446–445

Role LW, Kelly JP (1991) The brain stem: cranial nerve nuclei and the monoaminergic system. In: Kandel ER, Schwartz JH, Jessell TM (eds) Principles of neural science, 3rd edn. Elsevier Science, Amsterdam, pp 683–699

Rood MS (1954) Neurophysiological reactions as a basis for physical therapy. Phys Ther Rev 34 (9):444–449

Sahrman SA (1993) Movement as a cause of musculoskeletal pain. In: Singer KP (ed) Integrating approaches. Proceedings of the Eighth Biennial Conference of the Manipulative Physical Therapists Association of Australia. 24–27 November, Perth, pp 69–74

Silbernagl S, Despopoulos A (1983) Taschenbuch der Physiologie. Thieme, Stuttgart

Slater H, Wright A, Vicenzino B (1993) Physiological effects of the 'sympathetic slump' on peripheral sympathetic nervous system function. In: Singer KP (ed) Integrating approaches. Proceedings of the Eighth Biennial Conference of the Manipulative Physical Therapists Association of Australia. 24–27 November, Perth, pp 94–97

Slater H, Vicenzino B, Wright A (1994) 'Sympathetic slump': the effects of a novel manual therapy technique on peripheral sympathetic nervous system function. J Manual Manipulative Ther 2(4):156–162

Umphred DA (1995) Limbic complex. In: Neurological rehabilitation, 3rd edn. Mosby, St. Louis, pp 92–117

Vojta V (1981) Die zerebrale Bewegungsstörungen im Säuglingsalter, 3rd edn. Enke, Stuttgart

Wasserman K, Whipp BJ (1975) Exercise physiology in health and disease. Am Rev Res Dis 112:219–249

Zilles K, Rehkämper G (1994) Funktionelle Neuroanatomie, 2nd edn. Springer, Berlin Heidelberg New York

Zimmermann M (1995) Das somatoviszerale sensorische System. In: Schmidt RF, Thews G (eds) Physiologie des Menschen, 26th edn. Springer, Berlin Heidelberg New York, pp 216–235

3 Motor Learning

OBJECTIVES

By the end of this chapter the reader will be able to:
- Understand the difference between declarative and procedual learning
- Distinguish between the cognitive, associative, and autonomous stages of learning
- Apply the concept of motor learning in using the Swiss ball

It is ever more important for therapists to understand how humans learn best. Substantial research is currently being carried out in motor learning and its memory aspects. The limbic system underlines the importance of motivation and memory in the learning process, although other parts of the brain participate in learning; "knowing why," for example, involves the frontal lobe, while the cerebellum assists in conditioning. *Declarative learning* deals with facts and events – "knowing that" – while *procedural learning* involves "knowing how" (Winstein 1997, personal communication). For instance, knowing *that* one should get under a table during an earthquake can be attributed to declarative learning, while knowing *how* to get under the table involves procedural learning. Repetition of the skill may help to get there fast. In declarative thought there may be a strong emotional and judgmental component while procedural learning deals more with skill, habit, and stereotypic behavior (such as getting us in the morning from one place to another; Umphred 1995).

- Declarative learning ("knowing that"): facts, events
- Procedural learning ("knowing how"): skills, habits

Problem solving involves both declarative and procedural learning. For example, only when the patient understands *that* it is important to be able to walk to the bathroom will he be willing to consider *how* to achieve the skill of walking.

To be able to teach movements, therapists must understand how humans acquire new motor skills, which is defined as a task requiring voluntary movements to reach the goal. There are several stages in learning a new task.

3.1 Stages of Learning

Fitts and Posner (1967) describe three stages of learning – the cognitive, associative, and autonomous:

- In the *cognitive stage* many errors are made, and often the learner *requires external help* to correct an activity that was performed incorrectly, for example, mastering a simple task at the computer, such as typing a page.
- In the *associative stage* performance varies. The person makes fewer mistakes and *is capable of self-correction* of some of the mistakes by recognizing what is wrong. In writing a page on the computer the person may be able to begin editing independently.
- The *autonomous stage* is reached when writing a page becomes routine. The person can *automatically correct mistakes* without even thinking about what to do. When a patient is required to learn a new exercise the same stages of learning can be expected.

There are also *performance-related changes* in a number of dimensions of learning a motor skill (Magill 1989), including:
- Changes in achieving the goal of a skill
- Changes in error detection and correction capability
- Changes in movement efficiency
- Changes in coordination
- Changes in EMG pattern

All these dimensions of changes are well known to therapists and can be observed with patients. Motor learning in normal adults can occur over the entire range of movement complexity (Gottlieb et al. 1988).

> For therapists it is very important to understand how to help patients in acquiring new skills and relearning old skills: Should the therapist provide substantial feedback or only a little? Is it important for the patient to know the result of a movement that is performed?

3.2 Knowledge of Result, Knowledge of Performance

Knowledge of result has been studied by a number of researchers. Schmidt et al. (1989, 1990) and Salmoni et al. (1984) found that knowledge of result guides the subject forward during the early stage of learning, but that it may diminish the subject's ability to detect errors for the person may come to depend on the information given.

> Receiving less knowledge of result from external sources enhances motor skill learning because the person thus becomes self-correcting (Winstein and Schmidt 1990; Winstein 1991). In the early stage of practice the performer is driven to a goal response; in the later stage less frequent feedback enhances learning.

Winstein et al. (1994) also found that *frequent physical guidance* results in high on-target performance but in poor retention. Subjects who received less frequent knowledge of result while learning a task, and who therefore had to learn from their own mistakes had much better retention. Kernodle and Carlton (1992) provided learners with cues to focus their attention on the relevant aspects of *knowledge of performance*, thus helping them to distinguish between what to do and how to do it.

3.3 Feedback

Studies of *instantaneous feedback* and learning have found that it may be advantageous to let subjects estimate their own errors before feedback is given (Swinnen et al. 1990). In this way the cerebellum is self-correcting and learns to refine the motor program. Feedback provides knowledge, motivation, and reinforcement (Fitts and Posner 1967). This applies to (a) *intrinsic feedback*, which is the natural feedback from the body (by feeling and seeing) about the rate of movement and location and (b) feedback from external sources, called *augmented feedback*. Knowledge of performance is an example of augmented feedback which comes from a source external to the person's own sensory system. *Augmented sensory feedback* uses an external device to augment sensory feedback that is already available (Magill 1993).

Transfer of learning is the application of learning achieved in one task setting to another task (Schmidt 1991). This can mean initially breaking a task into separate elements to make it easier to learn and to facilitate the transfer to a more complex movement.

3.4 Clinical Applications: Examples

Knowledge of the processes involved in motor learning is helpful when using the Swiss ball.

> In patients who cannot perform the task as a total program, transfer of learning is applied, and a complicated skill such as walking is first broken down into simpler tasks.

The patient can learn alternate movements of the legs while lying on his back (e.g., see the exercise "Perpetual Motion," Sect. 9.22) without having to worry about trunk control or speed of movement. The patient then can be asked to move his legs alternately at a gait speed.

The normal walking speed of adults is approximately 82 m per minute; on a smooth surface this corresponds to a cadence of some 117 steps per minute for women and 111 for men (Perry 1992). The mean adult cadence is 113 steps per minute. Later the skill in moving the legs alternately at a gait speed while lying on the back can be transferred to moving the legs alternately at a gait speed while sitting on the Swiss ball.

The patient can now learn how to keep the pelvis, trunk, and head in good upright posture and move the arms while bouncing on the ball and taking steps on the same spot at gait speed. Finally these skills are transferred to walking upright in the room at gait speed.

Good strength of the muscles and balance and coordination are required to master the task, and the ball provides the patient and therapist with feedback for knowledge of performance and of the result. It is not necessary for the therapist to tell the patient what he cannot do. Using the ball, the therapist can help the patient find out for himself what he can and cannot do and give cues or demonstrate how to perform a task. The patient himself then can exercise at home and learn the skill.

A patient in supine position, moving his leg on a Swiss ball in a straight line, can see how well he is doing especially when visual cues are given. Since the patient must also watch that the leg does not "fall" off the ball while moving it, another dimension is added, and more attention is required.

The therapist can also demonstrate how to perform the exercise or provide augmented feedback by stating that "the ball is not rolling in a straight line yet," or "watch the dot on the knee" or by placing a mirror in front of the patient when he is sitting on the ball as long as the patient has the visual spatial skill.

At a later point the patient should be able to perform the exercise without visual feedback. The elasticity and the mobility of the ball require constant subconscious or conscious vigilance. Attention and concentration are also elicited. The muscles readjust automatically to the constantly changing demands.

3.5 Plasticity of the Brain

Plasticity of the brain is the basis of restoring function after a stroke (Mauritz 1994), and recovery from a stroke can continue for months or years (Bach-Y-Rita 1987). It is the plasticity of the brain which causes dynamic reorganization and adaptation to new circumstances, permitting enduring functional changes to take place. Behavioral factors influencing the plasticity/recovery of motor function include (Winstein 1995):

- Active participation
- Meaningful goals
- Practice (skill acquisition)

It is important to incorporate *active problem solving* into treatment when the patient is able to do so. Unmasking of unused synapses can become a mechanism of neural plasticity (Mauritz 1994; Jacobs and Donoghue 1991). Uncrossed ipsilateral pyramidal tracts and bilateral tracts originating in the primary motor cortex are also important for the recovery of function (Mauritz 1994).

> Sprouting from axons may contribute to the recovery by forming new connections (Mauritz 1994).

Some pyramidal and especially nonpyramidal fibers from the brain stem are likely to contribute redundancy for motor control, which may account for persons with hemiplegia regaining modest arm function and sufficient use particularly of their antigravity muscles on the paretic side to advance the leg for walking (Dobkin 1993).

The importance of the ipsilateral corticospinal system in the recovery is stressed by Miller Fisher (1991), who describes two patients with pure motor hemiplegia who had regained strength in the affected limbs after a subsequent motor stroke on the opposite side of the brain. The second stroke resulted in bilateral paralysis, destroying the gains achieved after the first stroke. It is currently thought that specific forms of intervention during learning can facilitate positive plasticity of the damaged brain (Winstein 1995).

> Practice can bring relatively permanent changes in behavior requiring different processes (Winstein 1995).

Learning has many facets, and much more research is required to understand the extent to which various areas of the CNS participate in the process. In applying concepts of motor learning to patients it is important to note both their emotional state and their ability to process and retain information. The therapist must always consider how the multiple systems are inter-acting.

> Therapists can enhance *procedural learning* by including many repeti-tions, which leads to skill acquisition, especially when the same task is varied in its execution. *Declarative learning* is achieved when the patient actively participates in the problem-solving aspect.

> The Swiss ball is a useful tool because it supplies a motivational link and can be used both by the patient and by the therapist for the solv-ing of problems. The ball enables the therapist to break a task down and allows the patient to practice what he is capable of toward achieving his goal by understanding that certain exercises must be carried out to achieve the functional goal set by patient and therapist.

References

Bach-Y-Rita P (1987) Process of recovery from stroke. In: Brandstater ME, Basmajian JV (eds) Stroke rehabilitation. Williams & Wilkins, Baltimore, pp 80–108

Dobkin BH (1993) Neuroplasticity – key to recovery after central nervous system injury. West J Med 159:56–60

Fitts PM, Posner MI (1967) Human performance. Brooks/Cole, Belmont

Gottlieb GL, Corcos DM, Jaric S, Agarwal GC (1988) Practice improves even the simplest movements. Exp Brain Res 73:436–440

Jacobs KM, Donoghue JP (1991) Reshaping the cortical motor map by unmasking latent in-tracortical connections. Sci 251:944–947

Kernodle MW, Carlton LG (1992) Information feedback and the learning of multiple degree-of-freedom activities. J Motor Behav 24(2):187–196

Magill RA (1989) Motor learning: concepts and applications, 3rd edn. Brown, Dubuque

Magill R (1993) Augmented feedback in skill acquisition. In: Singer RN, Murphey M, Ten-nant LK (eds) Handbook of research on sport psychology. Macmillan, New York, pp 193–212

Mauritz KH (1994) Rehabilitation nach Schlaganfall. Kohlhammer, Stuttgart

Miller Fisher C (1991) Concerning the mechanism of recovery in stroke hemiplegia. J Can Sci Neuro 19(1):57–63

Perry J (1992) Gait analysis. Slack, Thorofare

Salmoni AW, Schmidt RA, Walter CB (1984) Knowledge of results and motor learning: a re-view and critical reappraisal. Psychol Bull 95(3):355–386

Schmidt RA (1991) Motor learning and performance. Human Kinetics, Rawdon

Schmidt RA, Young DE, Swinnen S (1989) Summary knowledge of results for skill acquisi-tion. J Exp Psychol15(2):352–359

Schmidt RA, Lange C, Young DE (1990) Optimizing summary knowledge of results for skill learning Human Mov Sci 9:325–348

Swinnen SP, Nicholson DE, Schmidt RA, Shapiro DC (1990) Information feedback for skill acquisition: instantaneous knowledge of result degrades learning. J Exp Psy 16(4):706–716

Umphred DA (1995) Limbic complex. In: Neurological rehabilitation, 3rd edn. Mosby, St. Louis, pp 92–178

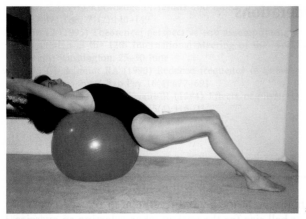

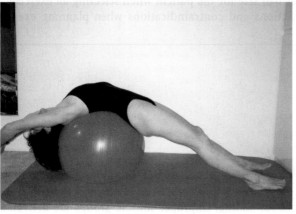

Fig. 4.1. a. Exercise performed incorrectly, because the feet are sliding. **b.** With traction, the exercise is performed correctly and looks harmonious.

floor between exercises. To *prevent cross-contamination* keep the same ball with the same patient and wash it before use.

It helps to place large Swiss balls on top of a hamper to clean them with water and soap (Fig. 4.2).

4.1.3 Pressure in the Ball

For all balance exercises the ball must be firmly inflated. This can be done best with a compressor, either at a gasoline station or with a small, commercially available compressor for inflating tires. A small vacuum cleaner with attachments for both exhaust and suction can be used to inflate and deflate the ball easily and quickly. Bicycle pumps generally lack the necessary volume and cannot compress the air in the ball. Mechanical pumps work if the

Fig. 4.2. Cleaning a Swiss ball on top of a linen hamper.

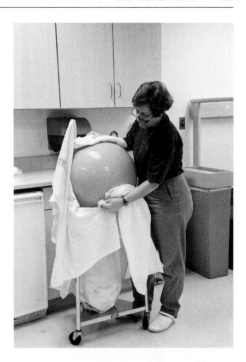

volume is sufficient. For comfort, deflate the ball some when positioning a patient prone over the ball. The pressure must be greater for heavier patients than for lighter ones. Most physical therapy departments offer Swiss balls of different sizes and pressures, which enables the therapist to choose the best ball for the intended exercises.

4.1.4 Size of the Ball

The patient's size does not determine which size of Swiss ball to use. At the most, it gives a general idea for the person who wants to sit on the ball.

Proportions and Body Build. It is recommended to look closely at the patient's proportions and body build (Klein-Vogelbach 1990a,b,c). The ball size must be selected on the basis of whether the patient has a long trunk and short legs, or a short trunk and long legs (Carrière and Felix 1993; Carrière 1993, 1996). When sitting on the Swiss ball, a long-legged person requires a larger ball (diameter 65 cm or more) than a short-legged one (55 cm diameter or less may be sufficient; Fig. 4.3).

Mobility. The therapist must observe whether the patient on a Swiss ball has the mobility to maintain a neutral spine easily when sitting with hips and knees at an angle of approximately 90°. In a neutral spine the pelvis, thorax,

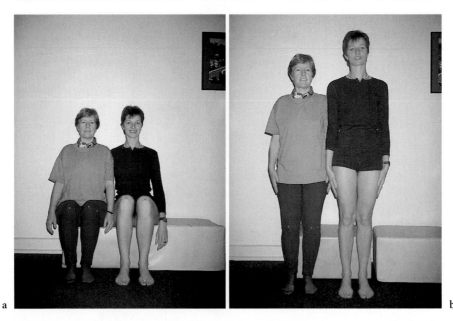

a   b

Fig. 4.3 a, b. Two persons of approximately the same size when sitting show different proportions when standing.

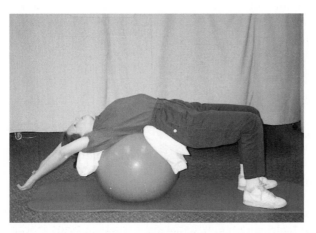

Fig. 4.4. Adaptating the size of the Swiss ball by increasing its diameter through the placement of pillows under the head and low back.

and head are aligned above one another, as three cubes stacked on top of each other. Only then are the natural curves of the spine maintained without difficulty or additional strain of the muscles. More than 90° mobility at the hip joints is necessary for the patient to sit up comfortably and without strain on the trunk muscles.

> The Swiss ball must be larger if the patient has decreased range of motion at one or both hip joints.

Reduced Mobility. A stiff spine or a spine with segments which show decreased mobility requires adaptation. If the therapist does not have access to a larger ball, a pillow can be used to accommodate for the lack of motion, increasing the diameter of the ball where needed (Fig. 4.4).

Lower Extremity Exercises in Supine or Prone. For exercises of the lower extremities when the patient is lying on his back (supine) or his stomach (prone), a smaller ball (45 or 55 cm) is usually sufficient.

4.2 Safety Conditions

> In using the Swiss ball the patient's safety should be the therapist's primary concern at all times!

The therapist must be aware of the patient's physical condition and any impairment in judgment or impulsiveness. Is the patient cautious, or a daredevil? Is he timid, or eager to try new exercises? Does the patient know about his sense of balance? How good is his body awareness? What preconditions may prevent the therapist from using the ball or require an exercise to be altered? During the physical therapist's initial evaluation of the patient it is important to know both the history of the patient's condition and the diagnosis provided by the physician in order to protect the patient from injuries.

Balance. Static and dynamic balance can be tested first in both sitting and standing with a stable base of support before challenging the patient's balance on the Swiss ball. One should distinguish between balance on a hard and on a soft surface since the first (e.g., sitting on a chair) requires somatosensory feedback while balance on a noncompliant surface such as a ball depends primarily on vestibular feedback. In the beginning the exercise can be performed close to a mat table or in the parallel bars if a patient tends to lean to one side. The patient's confidence is improved if he knows that he cannot "fall." In some patients with balance problems, a second person may be required to stand behind or next to the patient to provide assistance.

Body Awareness. Patients with decreased sensation on one or both sides of the body and decreased body awareness need to be watched closely. Mirrors and dots should be used to increase awareness and enable the patient to carry out the exercises safely if there are no visual-spatial deficits.

Use of Belt. A belt placed around the patient's waist helps the therapist physically to hold onto the patient until the patient finds his center of gravity. Initially the patient can keep his hands on the ball to decrease its mobility and can place his feet apart when sitting on the ball to increase the base of support.

Sandbags or Wedges, Stabilizers. Sandbags or wedges can be placed along the side of the ball to prevent it from rolling away (see Fig. 2.6a). Some companies provide a support base to be placed under the ball (e.g., Stabilizer by Sissel Orthopedic Products, Temecula, CA). Ledraplastic manufactures a Sit'n Gym, a ball with four spikes which keeps the ball from rolling away (Ball Dynamics International, Denver, CO)

PhysioRoll. The PhysioRoll, also made by Ledraplastic (Ball Dynamics, Denver, CO), is a double ball which rolls in two directions only. When a patient is learning to use the Swiss ball it may be safer to begin with the PhysioRoll because it has a wide base of support and functions similarly to training wheels on a bicycle, providing increased safety and instilling confidence in the patient's ability (Fig. 4.5).

Clothes and Shoes. It is important to wear proper clothes. "Slippery" pants or tops are not appropriate as they can cause the patient to slide off the ball and fall. Oversize clothes are also unsafe; they can become entangled or cause the patient to roll with the ball over his clothes, resulting in tripping or falling.

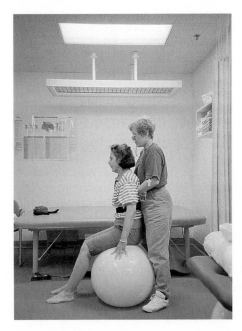

Fig. 4.5. Patient with transverse myelitis sitting on a PhysioRoll with a belt around her waist and a mirror in front of her for learning to maintain her balance in sitting.

Long Loose Hair. If not tied up, long loose hair can cause the patient to become entangled or roll over it.

Damaged Balls. Signs of damage, such as superficial cuts, can cause the ball to break at any time and are hazardous. Damaged balls should never be used with a patient.

> **Important: Do not try to repair a broken ball; get rid of it!**

Heat. Swiss balls expand when left in the sun or in a hot car and can burst. If kept in these environments, they should not be fully inflated to allow for the hot air to expand.

Overinflating of the Ball. Use only the recommended diameter when inflating a ball as it otherwise may burst.

Plugs. For additional safety some Swiss balls have long plugs which cannot be swallowed easily by children and are more difficult to remove.

Weight. Most Swiss balls can bear at least 200 kg weight. Check to be sure how much weight can be applied when working with a very heavy patient.

Space. Provide space and anticipate some of the difficulties which the patient may have when using the ball. Remove chairs and tables if necessary so that the patient can maneuver safely.

> **The best safety precaution is for the therapist to know the patient and the exercises well and to use common sense.**

4.3 Precautions, Contraindications

The best precaution is to use common sense.

Pain. Pain caused by exercises is a contraindication. The therapist must consider two causes of pain:
- The exercise is performed *incorrectly.*
- The exercise is performed *correctly but is not appropriate at this time for the patient.*

If careful observation leads to finding the cause, the patient can be instructed to perform the exercise correctly, and pain should thus cease. If the exercise causes pain although it is performed correctly, it needs to be abandoned and replaced by an exercise which the patient can perform without feeling pain. Since fear can also induce or intensify pain, therapists should avoid exercises which might do so.

> "Pain during an exercise can be a helpful warning to prevent something worse" – as Klein-Vogelbach taught in her classes on the Swiss ball – and therefore it should not be ignored.

Therapists must understand pain and interpret it correctly. Does it stem from an injury? Is it musculoskeletal in origin, or is it due to the stretching of tight muscles/tendons? Does it arise from fear and thus cause splinting? Adjustments must be made accordingly. If follow-through with exercises is expected from the patient, the exercises must not hurt.

> Pain is not a good motivator as no one would want to perform exercises which inflict pain.

Non-Weight-Bearing or Partial Weight-Bearing. A weight-bearing limitation of one or both lower extremities should prevent treatment in the sitting position, as the patient needs to bear weight on his legs if he loses his balance. However, a patient can exercise in supine position and place the ball under his leg (if there are no orthopedic/surgical contraindications) and perform exercises, enabling him to move without bearing the weight of the trunk or the extremity. Because the weight of the leg is supported by the ball, exercises can be carried out with reduced weight; the patient can move the leg without having to lift its weight.

Amputation. If one or both extremities are amputated, the patient's balance is greatly affected, and it may be unsafe to sit the patient on the Swiss ball. However, a patient with an amputated leg wearing a prosthesis may learn to balance his body when sitting on the ball. The therapist can use a belt and take other safety precautions when exercising with the patient. When a patient has an amputation of the upper extremity, balance is affected because the weight of the amputated arm is missing on one side. This must be considered.

Surgeries. Some surgeries may be a contraindication depending on how the exercise is performed; *the therapist needs to check with the physician.*

Shunts. When a ventricular-peritoneal shunt is present, there may be contraindications which should be checked with the surgeon. In the case of a newly placed shunt the patient may need to stay flat in the bed; more often his head is be elevated at least 30°.

Tubes, Monitors, Lines. Especially in the hospital therapists must know where tubes and lines come from and must check with the physician regarding what precautions to take. There may be contraindications for certain exercises and positions. For example, bending the hip with a femoral line in the groin certainly limits the degree to which the leg can be bent. A gastrostomy tube may prevent the therapist from putting the patient prone on the ball.

Respirator. In general a patient on a respirator can exercise with the Swiss ball, but of course the tubes should be watched and the exercises should not irritate the patient. Exercises must be selected carefully. Patients on a respirator may be critically ill, and Swiss ball exercises may be contraindicated. Check with the physician about precautions.

Seizures. If a patient with seizures is able to walk around without suffering seizures, and the colors of the ball do not irritate him, he can certainly use the Swiss ball for exercises. If the therapist knows that certain movements or movement speeds cause the patient problems, the exercises must be individualized to the patient's ability.

Decreased Balance and Body Awareness. Although decreased balance and body awareness of the patient must be considered for safety reasons, such factors are not a contraindication in general.

Geriatric Patients. In elderly patients with known osteoporosis *it is important to avoid falls.* A small ball may be most appropriate to encourage the patient to use it for exercising in bed but not for sitting on it. Use of the Swiss ball may be contraindicated in patients with advanced osteoporosis.

Pediatric Patients. *Supervise children at all times.* Do not leave a child alone with a ball that is too large. The patient may try to mount the ball, and fall.

References

Carrière B (1993) Swiss ball exercised. PT Magazine Phys Ther 9:92–100
Carrière B (1996) Therapeutic exercises and self-correction programs. In: Flynn T (ed) The thoracic spine and rib cage. Butterworth-Heinemann, Boston, pp 289–310
Carrière B, Felix L (1993) In consideration of proportions. PT Magazine Phys Ther 4:56–61
Klein-Vogelbach S (1990a) Functional kinetics: Springer, Berlin Heidelberg New York
Klein-Vogelbach S (1990b) Ballgymnastik zur Funktionellen Bewegungslehre, 3rd edn. Springer, Berlin Heidelberg New York
Klein-Vogelbach S (1990c) Functional kinetics: Swiss ball videotape. Springer, Berlin Heidelberg New York

5 Points of Observation

OBJECTIVES

By the end of this chapter the reader will be able to:
- Observe the contact points of the patient relative to the environment
- Judge the distribution of body weight which may affect the exercises
- Correct the performance of the exercise by changing the base of support
- Instruct correction of exercises by changing the body distances
- Recognize evasive movements by observation of critical points
- Understand how body proportions can affect the outcome of the exercises
- Vary exercises at hinged joints
- Correct evasive movements

To be able to correct exercises and adapt equipment to the patient's need the therapist *must develop keen observational skills*. Klein-Vogelbach (1990a,b,c) teaches the therapist to observe contact points both of the equipment with the environment and of the patient with the environment. In the following examples the floor serves as the environment; however, the same principle applies when the contact points are the mat table or, in some exercises, the wall.

5.1 Ball – Floor

When looking at the contact point between ball and floor, the therapist can determine whether the ball is properly inflated for the patient's size and weight and for the exercise intended.

> The ball moves more easily when there is less contact between ball and floor.

Greater inflation reduces the ball's base of support, and more equilibrium is required than on a soft ball, which increases the area of contact with the floor.

> With a soft, very compliant ball the patient may have only vision and vestibular input for balance; however, with a hard ball somatosensory input is probably also used.

The therapist can also observe whether the ball rolls in a straight line in the intended direction. When an exercise is difficult, the patient may "cheat" by changing the direction in which the ball is rolling or letting it roll when it is supposed to be stationary.

EXAMPLES

> *Figure 5.1.* Panel a. A patient lying prone over the Swiss ball walks forward on both hands until the feet are in the air, and the pelvis is on top of the ball. The therapist asks the patient to do a push-up. If done correctly, the shoulders are lowered in the direction of the hands while the ball remains stationary.
>
> Panel b. If the patient has any difficulties, the contact point between ball and floor moves away from the hands, making the exercise easier for the patient. This is the case as the shoulders move in the direction of the feet, and are no longer over the hands.
>
> Panel c. If the therapist wants to make the push-up very challenging, the patient can be asked not to move the hands on the floor while observing the ball moving closer to the hands when doing the push-up. The shoulders move in front of the hands.

5.2 Ball – Body

Again, by observing the contact points between the ball and the body the therapist is able to evaluate whether the exercise is being carried out as intended. Using the same example as in Fig. 5.1 of a push-up in prone-position over the ball, the therapist observes the patient "cheating" to make the exercise easier. The contact point between pelvis and ball changes and moves cranially, toward the abdomen. If the therapist wishes to make the same exercise more difficult, the contact point between ball and body must move more caudally, with the patient lying on the ball with his thighs.

> When sitting on the Swiss ball and bouncing up and down, the patient must maintain contact with the ball at all times; otherwise the ball may roll away and cause the patient to fall (unless the ball is in a Stabilizer).

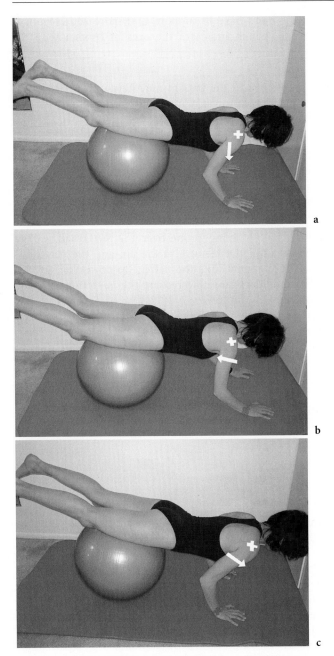

Fig. 5.1. a. Push-up with shoulder over the hand and pelvis on Swiss ball. **b.** The same exercise but with the ball moving cranially, making it easier for the patient. The shoulder is no longer over the hand but has moved backward. **c.** The same exercise but with the ball moving caudally, making the exercise more challenging. The shoulder now moves forward, increasing the load on the muscle triceps brachii.

It is also important to ensure that the patient sits on top of the center of the ball. Sitting off-center changes the movement of the ball since it begins to rotate when the contact point is more than 45° off-center (Klein-Vogelbach 1990b).

5.3 Body–Floor

Depending on the exercise, the contact point can remain stationary (in a constant location). Both the Swiss ball and the patient's feet remain on the same spot when bouncing. With other exercises the contact point between body and floor changes slightly, for example, when alternately lifting the legs while bouncing. With nonstationary (location-changing) exercises the contact point between body and floor changes completely (e.g., The "Sea Urchin," Sect. 9.14) For proper instruction of exercises, the therapist must know whether this contact point should change or not. If the traction on the mat/ floor is insufficient and the patient slides, the contact points change.

Small feet decrease the amount of contact with the floor and the base of support as well as the distance which the ball can roll.

5.4 Base of Support

The base of support (BOS) is determined by the contact which the ball has with the floor and the contact which the body has with the floor. A firm ball decreases the BOS and makes it more triangular than a soft ball.

> The BOS is the space between all the contact points.

This includes the feet when sitting on the ball. It is smaller when the feet are placed close together than when placed far apart. *The patient uses a BOS which makes him feel safe and able to do the exercise.* One can use a larger BOS when beginning to learn an exercise and decrease it when the patient is familiar with the exercise and ready to make the exercise more challenging.

The therapist can try to sit on the ball with the feet apart, close together, or on tip toes with one foot in front of the other and feel the increase of difficulty with each change. The effect of the BOS can be experienced when walking on the hands lying prone over a PhysioRoll or a ball, first with the feet apart, then close together or on a soft versus a firm ball. "Cheating" occurs over the BOS.

> If a patient seems to be carrying out an exercise easily when it should in fact be difficult, the therapist should look closely at the BOS.

The change in the BOS also alters the other contact points, and evasive movements can be observed at these other points of contact.

5.5 Bisecting Plane

The bisecting plane is an imaginary one which Klein-Vogelbach created for observation (1990a,b, 1991; Carrière 1993) when planning and adapting exercises. Imagine a vertical plane projected through the center of gravity of the body. It is over the BOS and at a right angle to the direction of movement. The bisecting plane divides the body into two halves and allows the therapist to assess the distribution of body weights. It must be regarded as though it were a scale with weights on either side (Fig. 5.2). The weights on the side of the direction of movement act to accelerate, while those on the other side act to decelerate, as a brake. If the lever on one side is too long/heavy compared to the counterweight, the patient shortens the lever, substitutes with muscles which are not intended to perform the work (substituting for weak muscles), or falls. The "Scale" exercise is a good example (Sect. 9.2).

> A patient with a long trunk, short legs, and weakened abdominal muscles uses one of the following substitutions or variations when sitting on top of the center of the ball to balance the body weight and avoid falling.

EXAMPLES

> *Figure 5.3.* Panel a. Good alignment of pelvis, trunk, and head, which requires activity of the abdominal muscles.
> Panel b. Anterior tilt of the pelvis, hyperextension of the low back, resulting in strain and pain to the low back muscles.
> Panel c. Anterior tilt of the pelvis, hyperextension of the low back, and a forward head, straining low back and neck muscles.
> Fig. 10.22a. and 11.27a. Posterior tilt of the pelvis, flexion of the trunk, and a forward head to shorten the long lever and to avoid straining the abdominal muscles.

When the arms are lifted above the head, the substitutions become more obvious because the lever is lengthened. This adds to the weight, which makes the exercise more difficult or even impossible for the patient.

EASY
long lower leg
short upper leg
long trunk

enough weight in front of the bisecting plane

DIFFICULT
short lower leg
long upper leg
short trunk

too much weight behind the bisecting plane

Fig. 5.2. The bisecting plane resembles to a scale, and the distribution of weights can be observed. (Drawing by Mary Sheh, from Carrière and Felix 1993, with kind permission from the publisher).

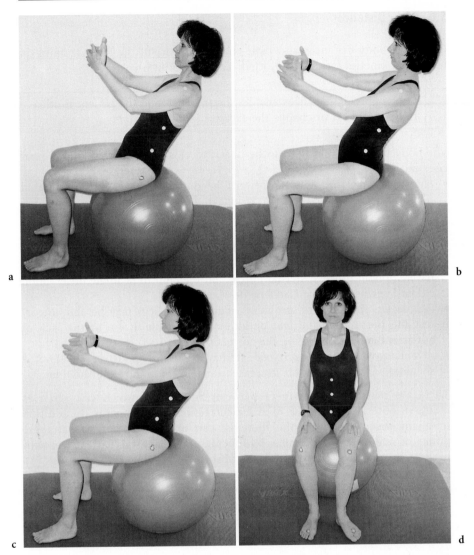

Fig. 5.3 a. Pelvis, trunk, and head in good alignment; the abdominal muscles are activated. **b.** Compensation with anterior tilt of the pelvis, causing increased strain to the low back. **c.** Compensation with anterior tilt of the pelvis and a forward head, causing strain to the low back and the neck. **d.** Body distances can be used for correction of posture and alignment; dots increase visual awareness.

Correction: Start the exercise slightly off center. Instead of weight bearing on the ischial tuberosity, the patient can bear his weight on the sacrum, making the weight distribution more equal. The therapist can also instruct the patient to keep his arms in front of the body, or on his lap.

5.6 Body Distances

Observing body distances and their changes is part of the basic training in functional kinetics (see Fig. 5.3, Klein-Vogelbach 1990a).

> Studying body distances enables the therapist and the patient to identify and correct or change the exercise.

The body distances that need to be observed closely when performing exercises include:

- *Sternal notch–chin.* With a forward head the distance between sternal notch and the tip of the chin is longer than in a neutral spine posture (with the pelvis, the trunk, and the head aligned).
- *Symphysis pubis–navel, navel–xiphoid process.* Sitting "slouched" with a posteriorly tilted pelvis and a flexed spine shortens these distances. Arching the back lengthens them. Dots can be placed on the symphysis pubis, navel, xiphoid process, sternal notch, and the chin to facilitate observation (Klein-Vogelbach 1990a; Carrière 1996).
- *Feet–knees.* Patients with problems aligning their legs may be able to correct the position of the feet or knees when made aware of the lack of alignment and by observing the correction (Fig. 5.3d).
- *Acromioclavicular joint–ear lobe.* It may be useful to detect an elevated shoulder or substitution for decreased range of motion of the shoulder.

There are many other distances between body parts which can serve as points of observation and be used for correction of movements. In addition to giving visual feedback, the therapist can provide tactile cues at these points of reference, for example, by touching or letting the patient feel with his own hands how to correct a faulty posture or alignment.

The advantage of using body distances for instruction and correction lies in the fact that the patient, unless he has a severe neurological defect, knows of these distances because they are part of his inborn kinesthetic awareness. It enables the patient to see and feel what changes are required to do exercises correctly, and how to improve posture and alignment.

5.7 Hinged Joints

Few therapist's are aware of the many possibilities for moving a hinged joint. Therapists most frequently move the distal lever, flexing the knee while sitting and moving the lower leg, pulling it toward the buttocks. However, the patient could also sit on a Swiss ball, keeping the heels on the floor, and roll the ball toward the feet. Clinical situations in which it may be helpful to move a hinged joint from the proximal lever or pivot point in order to flex the knee include:

- When the patient is *fearful* to move a joint
- When the patient has a *contracture*
- When the patient is using *evasive movements*
- To *detect errors* and give *precise instructions*

Klein-Vogelbach (1990a) describes ten possibilities for moving a hinged joint. At least five or six of these can be used with patients when performing exercises; the other four are normally used with a movement sequence such as kicking or throwing a ball or jumping. If there is a contracture or a limp, the therapist should observe the movement closely at both levers and the fulcrum to detect why the movement is faulty.

Hinged joints have a fulcrum point at which the movement takes place, and two levers.

> The amount of movement that takes place can be observed most easily at the most distal point of each lever.

If we imagine the knee joint as a fulcrum, the proximal lever P is the thigh and the distal lever D the lower leg. The most distant visible point on the proximal lever is near the trochanter, on the distal lever, the lateral or medial malleolus.

There are five ways to *decrease the amount of movement without moving the fulcrum,* and five possibilities for movement of the fulcrum, for example, when flexing the knee:

1. The proximal lever P moves toward the distal lever D. This means that the malleolus and the knee do not move in space while the thigh is flexing at the knee joint (Fig. 5.4 a, b).
2. The distal lever D moves toward the lever P. The trochanter and the fulcrum knee remain stationary in space, and the lower leg flexes the knee.

EXAMPLES

Lying prone and lifting the foot and lower leg to bend the knee.

3. The knee does not move while the proximal lever P and distal lever D move toward each other.

EXAMPLES

Standing on hands and knees, lifting the heels toward the hips while rocking backward moving the hips to the direction of the heels.

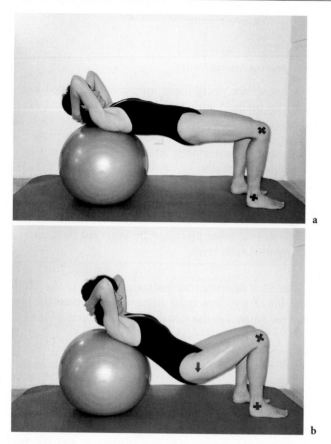

Fig. 5.4a, b. Starting and end positions of proximal lever P moving toward distal lever D; fulcrum remains stationary in space.

4, 5. Both levers move in the same direction, but one more than the other.

> **EXAMPLES**
>
> Imagine kneeling on hands and knees. While lowering the hips to the floor the knees can bend. The thigh and lower leg move in a circular motion in the same direction. Increased knee flexion occurs when the lower leg moves more in space than the thigh.

During evasive movements, as frequently seen in patients with contractures, the two levers of a hinged joint move an equal amount (Fig. 5.5).

The five possibilities with movement of the fulcrum are:

6. The proximal lever P and the fulcrum knee move, and the most distal point of the lever D remains almost stationary (Fig. 5.6a).
7. The distal lever D and the fulcrum move, and the point of lever P furthest away from the joint is almost stationary (Fig. 5.6b, c).

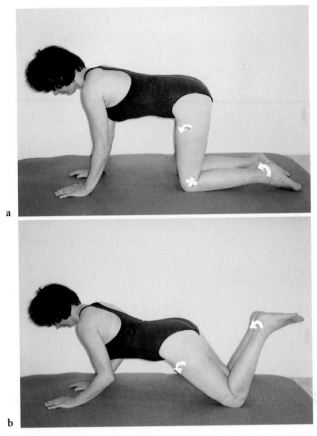

Fig. 5.5 a, b. Starting and end positions while standing on hands and knees; the two levers P and D move in the same direction, and the fulcrum remains on the floor.

8. Both levers P and D move toward each other, and the fulcrum moves (Fig. 5.7).

9, 10. These can be observed during a sequence of movement, for example, a somersault forward and back. The two levers move in a circular motion in the same direction, the fulcrum also moves, and one lever moves more than the other, increasing flexion of the knee.

Therapists can also observe, for example, when extending the flexed arm, that the fulcrum remains stationary when only the forearm is moved while extending the elbow. The direction of this movement is semicircular. If the movement pattern is a straight line, the fulcrum must also move.

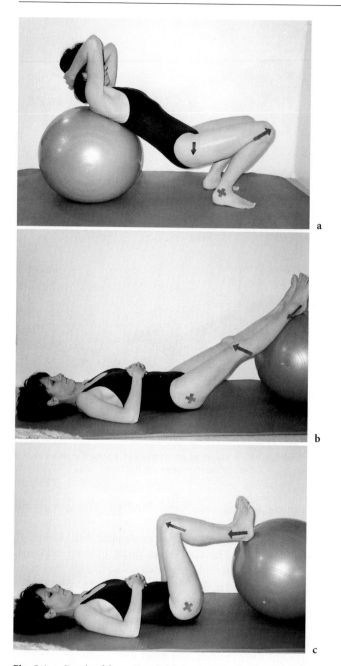

Fig. 5.6. a. Proximal lever P and fulcrum move, the most distal point of lever D remains stationary. **b, c.** Distal lever D and the fulcrum move; the most distal point of the lever P remains stationary.

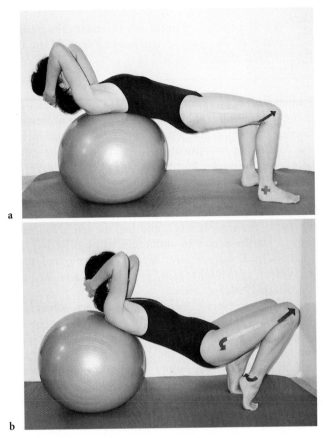

Fig. 5.7 a, b. Starting and end positions. Both levers P and D and the fulcrum move.

5.8 Continuing Movement and Buttressing

> When observing movement, it is very important to identify where the movement begins and where it ends. How does the first movement impulse continue and end? Which joints are involved, which direction does the movement take? Do all joints and levers between the initial impulse and the end of the movement participate? Does the movement remain in the same plane of movement? How far should the movement go?

The therapist must observe the movement keenly. An evasive movement secondary, for example, to a contracture or to pain results in one or several joints not participating in the continuing movement.

A patient with a painful left shoulder. The patient flexes the spine laterally to the right to compensate for lack of abduction movement in the left shoulder joint.

Proper instructions are necessary to correct this faulty continuing movement; the therapist can instruct a countermovement of the right arm. Abducting the right arm causes a second movement impulse and neutralizes the continuing movement of the left arm if the movement amount and the speed are the same. The therapist *activates a counterweight* (the right arm) to move in the opposite direction (referred to in functional kinetics as *activated passive buttressing*).

The therapist can also create an awareness of the faulty movement pattern by letting the patient touch and feel the left shoulder move and then instruct him to lift the arm into abduction without letting the shoulder move closer to the ear. If only *muscle activity* is generated to prevent the continuing movement, *active buttressing* is the term used in functional kinetics (Klein-Vogelbach 1990a,b,c, 1991).

When performing Swiss ball exercises, observation of the continuing movement helps the therapist to prevent or correct errors. The exercise "Hula-Hula" (Sect. 9.8) serves as an example. Without proper instructions the lateral movement of the hip continues into the trunk and causes it to lean to the side. With proper instruction (e.g., the frontotransverse diameter of the thorax remains stable in space while the pelvis moves side to side) the patient limits the lateral flexion to the lumbar region.

References

Carrière B (1996) Therapeutic exercises and self-correction programs. In: Flynn T (ed) The thoracic spine and rib cage. Butterworth-Heinemann, Boston, pp 289–310
Carrière B, Felix L (1993) In consideration of proportions. PT Magazine Phys Ther 4:56–61
Klein-Vogelbach S (1990a) Functional kinetics: Springer, Berlin Heidelberg New York
Klein-Vogelbach S (1990b) Ballgymnastik zur Funktionellen Bewegungslehre, 3rd edn. Springer, Berlin Heidelberg New York
Klein-Vogelbach S (1990c) Functional kinetics: Swiss ball videotape. Springer, Berlin Heidelberg New York
Klein-Vogelbach S (1991) Therapeutic exercises in functional kinetics. Springer, Berlin Heidelberg New York

6 Exercise Terminology and Muscle Activity

OBJECTIVES

By the end of this chapter the reader will be able to:
- Understand functional kinetics terminology
- Recognize the various states of muscle activity
- Modify exercises with the purpose of changing the muscle activity
- Apply the principle of active/reactive muscle training
- Determine actio-reactio and conditio-limitatio of exercises

Awareness of muscle activity is important when planning and analyzing exercises. The therapist must select the exercise. Should the exercise be easy or difficult, performed consciously or subconsciously, with or against gravity? Should body weights be used or free weights? Klein-Vogelbach (1990a,b,c, 1991) was a master at observing movements and modifying exercises to fit the patient's needs. To enable her students to learn her skills, she developed an exercise terminology which is familiar to all functional kinetics instructors and students.

6.1 Exercise Terminology

6.1.1 Body Segments

Klein-Vogelbach (1990a) describes the five following body segments as functional units:
- Head and neck
- Arms and shoulder girdle
- Thoracic spine
- Lumbar spine and pelvis
- Legs

In an upright neutral posture the head and neck, the lumbar spine, and the pelvis require potential mobility, while the thoracic spine requires dynamic stabilization. There is close interdependence of these states of activity. The arms and the shoulder girdle need a dynamically stable trunk to move freely in an open kinetic chain.

> The head and neck require a stable base as well. During walking the weight-bearing leg is in a closed kinetic chain requiring dynamic stability, while the other leg is potentially mobile in a open kinetic chain.

6.1.2 Potential Mobility

> Standing in a neutral posture with pelvis, trunk, and head aligned, potential mobility is the *readiness of muscles to adapt to constant changes in positions of the joints in reaction to changes in equilibrium* (Klein-Vogelbach 1990a). This readiness must be greater when the base of support (BOS) is smaller. Potential mobility requires good mobility of joints, normal strength of muscles, and a stable base. Faulty movement patterns can develop, and the ability to move is decreased if potential mobility is lost.

6.1.3 Dynamic Stabilization

Dynamic stabilization is *fixation of one or several joints of a body segment or parts thereof through muscle activity.* Dynamic stability is maintained during the movement of these joints in space and when adding weights (body or free weights). Inability to move the stable trunk in space without losing stability usually increases muscular and ligamentous strain.

> **EXAMPLES**
>
> Leaning forward with a poorly dynamically stabilized spine often results in low back or neck strain. The potential mobility of the low back and pelvis is lost, and the ability to move and adjust to changes is decreased.
> Sit slouched and feel the change of posture and the decrease in movement of the spine. The neck and low back have lost their potential mobility. The dynamic stability is restored when sitting upright, allowing head and trunk to move freely.

6.2 Variations of Muscle Activity

6.2.1 Parking Function

In the parking function *muscle activity is low and economical.* There is just enough muscle activity to maintain the position of the body without causing any strain. Only the weight of a body segment or part thereof exerts pressure

Fig. 6.1. Parking function. The legs rest with their own weight on the floor.

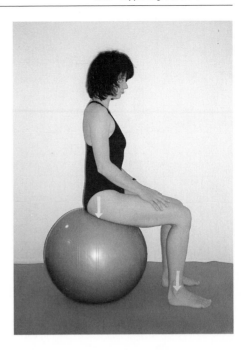

onto the BOS. It is a closed chain position without cocontraction, for example, of the lower extremity muscles when sitting on a Swiss ball or on a chair. A parking position is used to start an exercise, for example, when sitting in a neutral spine position on a ball, with the legs flexed at 90° to ankles, knees, and hips. The activity of the quadriceps muscles is low (Fig. 6.1).

6.2.2 Supporting Function

Muscle activity is high and economical. It is a closed chain activity with cocontraction of the muscles exerting pressure on the BOS. When sitting on a ball and leaning forward, the pressure under the feet and the activity of the quadriceps muscles increases. When increasing the pressure over the feet by decreasing the pressure of the buttocks on the ball, the activity of the quadriceps further increases because the BOS and the bisecting plane changes. Consequently part of the thigh, pelvis, and most of the trunk are weights which must be held by the muscles of the legs (Fig. 6.2). The muscle activity begins distally: the lower leg must be stabilized over the foot, the thigh on the lower leg, etc.

Supporting function is very useful when working on dynamic stabilization. This means that a body segment or parts thereof are stabilized with muscle activity during movement or when adding weights (body or free weights).

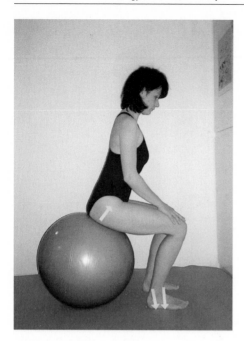

Fig. 6.2. Support function. The legs must support the weight of the trunk, head, and arms.

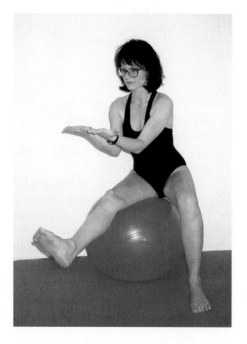

Fig. 6.3. Free play function. Most of the muscle activity is on top of the extremity.

When changing from upright sitting to a standing position, the muscle activity changes from parking to supporting function.

6.2.3 Free-Play Function

Suspension of an extremity from the body in an open kinetic chain with some activity directed against gravity is referred to in functional kinetics terms as *free play*. Muscle activity is predominantly on the upper side of the extremity, preventing its fall. Muscle activity is greater when the extremity is extended in a more horizontal position because more body weights must be held against gravity. *The muscle activity extends from proximal to distal.*

EXAMPLES

An arm in a free-play function: the upper arm is held by the muscles of the shoulder girdle, the forearm by the muscles of the upper arm, and the hand by the forearm. Subtle changes of muscle activity can be initiated by changing the position; the activity is on the top of the extremity.

Extend one arm externally rotated in the shoulder with supination of the forearm and palm up. Palpate the activity of the biceps brachii muscle, which is greater than that of the muscle triceps brachii. When turning the arm internally at the shoulder and pronating the extended arm, the muscle triceps brachii has a palpable greater activity than the biceps muscle.

When the weight of the suspended extremity is too great, it usually results in a compensatory mechanism, for example, leaning the trunk backward while lifting forward the extended arms with weights (Carrière 1996). This is an adjustment to the distribution of weight on each side of the bisecting plane as described in Chap. 5. Walking entails a constant change from a closed kinetic chain and supporting function to an open kinetic chain and free-play function. In the exercise "Cocktail Party," one leg is in support function and the other in free-play function (Fig. 6.3).

Pushing off from a surface is also a change from a support to a free play function.

6.2.4 Bridging Activity

Imagine a bridge construction with pillars on both ends. A similar construction exists when kneeling on hands and knees, with the legs and arms acting as pillars, and the trunk as the bridge. If the stomach sags, the low back hangs on the pelvis, and the upper and middle part of the back on the shoulder girdle. Activating the abdominal muscles underneath the bridge against gravity to prevent the bridge from sagging is called a bridge activity. When lying prone over a ball, the arms serve as two pillars and the Swiss ball as the other pillar. The activity of the muscles of the trunk, especially the abdominal muscles, is increased because the ball is labile and the activity more challenging.

> The size of the bridge and the amount of contact of the pillars with the floor determines how difficult the exercise is. This also depends on the strength and skill of the muscles involved (Fig. 6.4).

A quadriceps muscle able to lift some free weights concentrically in an open kinetic chain may have difficulty contracting concentrically in a bridging activity.

> **EXAMPLES**
> Lie prone with the knee bent and the foot resting on a 45-cm (yellow) Swiss ball. Move the knee into extension and lower it into flexion again in a straight line to feel the skill required to do so. Imagine a patient who has had knee surgery affecting his proprioception or a person with mild spasticity who is able to extend the flexed knee in an open chain. These patients may have great difficulty or be unable to activate their quadriceps in a bridging activity (see Fig. 11.5).

6.2.5 Hanging Activity

Suspension of body segments or parts thereof from another part of the body or an external object is called hanging activity. Muscle activity extends from distal to proximal, that is, from the source of suspension toward the center of the body. The joints below the suspension are distracted. Body weight must be considered when the entire body is hanging from a bar in an open kinetic chain. Because of the direction of the muscle activity the weight of the pelvis and legs must be held by the low back muscles, which is a strain to the back. The patient instead could sit on a Swiss ball, face and hold on to the stall bars above the head, roll the ball away from the stall bars, and keep the feet on the floor. Holding onto the therapist, the patient can be in control, distracting his back and his shoulders (Fig. 6.5). To limit the distraction to the low back the therapist can hold the patient on the trunk.

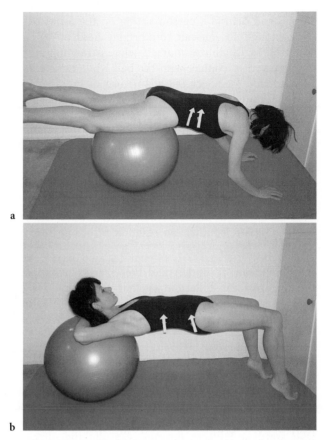

a

b

Fig. 6.4a,b. Bridging activity. **a.** Prone on Swiss ball, abdominal strengthening in bridging activity. **b.** Supine on Swiss ball, hip extensors stabilize against gravity.

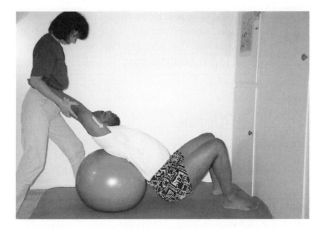

Fig. 6.5. Hanging activity, distracting the back – holding on to the physical therapist.

EXAMPLES

Stand behind a person sitting on the Swiss ball. Bend your knees just enough so you can comfortably hold on to each side of the person's thorax. Stabilize yourself while straightening your knees. Leave the person in contact with the ball while he is rocking it gently from side to side (see Sect. 9.8 adaptation of the "Hula-Hula"). The distraction is limited to the area between your hands and the ball and is usually very comfortable to the patient.

6.3 Primary Movement, Actio–Reactio

Actio is the primary movement toward the goal, and *reactio* is the automatic equilibrium reaction resulting from the actio.

It is important to understand these terms when planning exercises because the therapist must decide whether the corrective exercise should be done consciously, or giving an instruction which results in an automatic use of the muscles (Klein-Vogelbach 1990a,b,c, 1991; Carrière 1993, 1996).

EXAMPLES

The patient can be instructed to perform a quadriceps set (tighten the quadriceps), which is a very direct instruction. This may not work, for example, if the patient fears using his quadriceps. The therapist then has many other choices to recruit the quadriceps reactively.
Sit on a Swiss ball and decrease the weight on the ball by leaning forward and lifting the buttocks slightly; alternatively, sit upright and move the ball as close as possible to the feet. A quadriceps activation results. Sit cross-legged on a Swiss ball and push the toes into the ground.
Each time the quadriceps muscles are activated as a result of another instruction, automatically and perhaps subconsciously. The body must react to the changes in the BOS and distribution of body weights and regain the state of equilibrium (reactive muscle training).

6.4 Conditio–Limitatio

The terms conditio and limitatio were coined by Klein-Vogelbach (1990a,b,c, 1991) for the purposes of instruction and analyzing movements.

Conditios, which are part of the actio, are verbal instructions given for the exercise to be carried out as intended.

One or more conditios are necessary depending on the difficulty of the exercise and the awareness and ability of the patient.

> *Limitatio* is the goal to be achieved by the reactio (e.g., stabilizing muscle activity, limiting the primary movement, achieving the ideal speed of movement).

There are three kind of conditios:

1. The conditio of *maintaining the body distances* (see Sect. 5.6). This results in a dynamic stabilization because muscles must hold the weight of body parts. The exercise "Scale" (Sect. 9.2) serves as an example. The actio in this exercise is to roll the Swiss ball toward the feet without increasing the weight over the feet. The conditio given to maintain the body distance navel–xiphoid results in the limitatio of dynamic stabilization of the trunk. Without this conditio the trunk probably would flex, the abdominal muscles would not be challenged, and the trunk not be stabilized.
2. The conditio concerning *relative or absolute fixed spatial points*. In the above exercise the therapist asks the patient to maintain the frontotransverse axis through the thorax fairly stable in space (relative fixed spatial point). It moves slightly up and down in space but should not move forward and back, since the ball should roll under the trunk and not move the trunk forward and back. The toes are an absolute fixed spatial point; they do not leave the floor at all when rolling the Swiss ball toward the heels. Moving in the other direction, the heels remain on the floor and are an absolute fixed spatial point. These conditios result in limiting the primary movement (limitatio).
3. The conditio concerning the *speed of movement*. The limitatio is to achieve the ideal speed, that is, the speed at which the patient can best perform the exercise. In many exercises the desired speed is the speed of gait, approximately 120 times per minute. For the "Scale" Klein-Vogelbach considers the ideal speed of leaning the trunk forward and back to be approximately 40 times per minute (Klein-Vogelbach 1990b).

Conditios serve to achieve economical movement and for the patient to perform the exercises correctly. The limitatio is not important for the patient but helps the therapist to determine what to achieve with the exercise, and to observe whether the exercise is carried out as intended.

References

Carrière B (1993) Swiss ball exercises. PT Magazine Phys Ther 9:92–100
Carrière B (1996) Therapeutic exercises and self correction programs. In: Flynn T (ed) The thoracic spine and ribcage. Butterworth-Heinemann, Boston, pp 289–310
Klein-Vogelbach S (1990a) Functional kinetics. Springer, Berlin Heidelberg New York

Klein-Vogelbach S (1990b) Ballgymnastik zur Funktionellen Bewegungslehre, 3rd edn. Springer, Berlin Heidelberg New York

Klein-Vogelbach S (1990c) Functional kinetics: Swiss ball videotape. Springer, Berlin Heidelberg New York

Klein-Vogelbach S (1991) Therapeutic exercises in functional kinetics. Springer, Berlin Heidelberg New York

7 Planning of Exercises, Screening, Evaluation, and Treatment

OBJECTIVES

By the end of this chapter the reader will be able to use the Swiss ball to:
- Screen/evaluate and treat strength and mobility
- Identify and treat alignment deficits
- Recognize problems resulting from muscle tonus impairments
- Screen/evaluate and treat balance deficits
- Identify and treat some neurotension problems

7.1 Evaluation

Patients who come to a therapist with a problem must receive a thorough evaluation before treatment begins. How the evaluation is conducted and what it includes depends on the patient's diagnosis and the therapist's background. Many different approaches are available for evaluating the patient's problems (e.g., Maitland 1986, 1992; Klein-Vogelbach 1990a; Bobath 1978; Butler 1991; Flynn 1996; Janda 1991, 1994a).

While the medical diagnosis of the patient indicates which systems in the body may be affected with pathology or disease, the therapist should not rely on the medical diagnosis alone.

> Patients with a neurological problem may also have muscle weakness from nonuse or disuse.
> Likewise, a patient with an orthopedic problem may also have neuromuscular deficits which must also be recognized and taken into consideration. That is, a patient's functional impairments/disabilities reflect the interaction of all systems within and surrounding the organism.

A new pathological condition interacting with an existing problem may create greater impairments than originally anticipated. Similarly, those systems which easily compensate for the breakdown of others may create less disability from a functional measurement than anticipated.

> For example, *approximately 10%–15% of children have minimal cere-*
> *bral dysfunction*, the symptoms of which are often hidden in adults.
> When an injury such as a simple strain or fracture occurs, minimal
> cerebral dysfunction can cause poor compensatory mechanisms, re-
> sulting in slower recovery and requiring more intensive therapy than
> initially expected (Janda 1994b).

The Swiss ball can serve as a tool to help evaluate both muscle weakness and
neurological deficit. Isolated muscles can be assessed in some instances, but
the evauluation is usually more global as numerous muscles participate in
the task. The therapist begins to recognize the patient's problem but may require specific assessments and detailed manual muscle testing to complete
the evaluation (e.g., Kendall 1993; Daniels and Worthingham 1986; Clarkson
and Gilewich 1989; Travell and Simons 1983, 1992; Janda 1994a).

> *Caution*: If the therapist notices abnormal programming during the
> evaluation, she should use other methods for evaluation and treat-
> ment, which may or may not mean a change in the suggested activity.

When testing muscle strength, the therapist should consider the following:
- Which body parts become a *weight* and must be lifted.
- How *body proportions* and muscle bulk affect performance during a test.
- How the *plane and the axis of the movement* are oriented in space.
- Whether the muscle is *loaded in a concentric, eccentric, or isometric man-
  ner.*

> Muscles fulfill their anatomical function when used concentrically as
> the muscle shortens and acts as a lifter.
> When a muscle lengthens and acts as a brake, the activity is ec-
> centric, while the activity of a muscle is considered isometric when
> movement is prevented (Klein-Vogelbach 1990a).

Muscles can move without having to lift only if their axis of movement is
spatially vertical and the plane in which the movement takes place is spatially horizontal (Klein-Vogelbach 1990a). The Swiss ball can be used to reduce the weight of the body segment or part thereof if the movement takes
place in a vertical plane and the axis of movement is spatially horizontal.
When evaluating strength, one should not forget that there is less substitution if the weight of the body segment or part thereof which normally must
be lifted is resting on a Swiss ball. Therapists must always remember that
muscles work in synergic patterns related to a functional task.

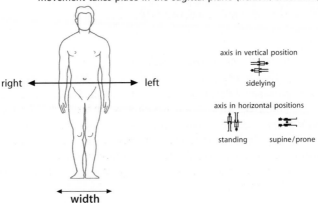

FRONTO-SAGITTAL-AXIS
Movement takes place in the transverse plane
(rotation)

up

length

down

axis in vertical position

standing

axis in horizontal positions

sidelying   supine/prone

SAGITTO-TRANSVERSE-AXIS
Movement takes place in the frontal plane
(abduction/adduction)

forward   backward

depth

axis in vertical position

supine/prone

axis in horizontal positions

standing   sidelying

FRONTO-TRANSVERSAL-AXIS
Movement takes place in the sagittal plane (flexion/extension)

right   left

axis in vertical position

sidelying

axis in horizontal positions

standing   supine/prone

width

Fig. 7.1. For the axes of movement, one vertical and two horizontal positions are possible in space. (Drawing by Mary Sheh).

Thus, when using the balls to grade strength and allow for active muscle synergic interaction, the therapist must remember at some time to transfer the ball activity to a specific functional activity.

Figure 7.1 is intended help the therapist recognize the position of axis and planes in space.

7.2 Muscle Strength and Range of Motion

Muscle Grading

Muscle grading in this chapter is based on the widely used scale of the Medical Research Council (1978; see also Florence et al. 1992), which ranges from 0 (no contraction) to 5 (normal muscle power):

0. No contraction
1. Flicker or trace of contraction
2. Active movement, with gravity eliminated
3. Active movement, against gravity
4. Active movement against gravity and resistance
5. Normal power

When a patient displays difficulties during screening/evaluation, the test position becomes an exercise for the patient to practice at home. "It is hard to do the exercise," one teenage patient repeatedly told me, but then she found satisfaction in returning a week later and showing off what she had not been able do previously. The feedback which the ball provides is a useful tool. Examples are provided below of how to screen muscle strength and range of motion (ROM) and to recognize substitution.

Comparing Muscle Strength (Hip Extensor Muscles)

With normal strength one hip can lift the pelvis and the other leg, as demonstrated in the exercise "Perpetual Motion" (Sect. 9.22; Klein-Vogelbach 1990b,c). Being able to feel for himself which side of the body lifts more easily motivates the patient, and the knowledge of result provides him with feedback when exercising. Both hands should be placed on the mat near the hips to stabilize the trunk and increase the base of support (BOS).

Patients with a muscle strength of 3/5 or greater are able to extend and lift both hips against gravity.

EXAMPLES

Figure 7.2. A patient with muscular dystrophy affecting the shoulder girdle demonstrates his inability to raise his arms while he is able to extend his hips in supine position. The bridging position makes it easy to test the strength of the hip extensor muscles and to compare the strength of the trunk of both sides of the body.

While the patient is bridging, the therapist can push the ball gently side to side and ask the patient to resist the movement. This demonstrates differences in strength on the two sides of the trunk.

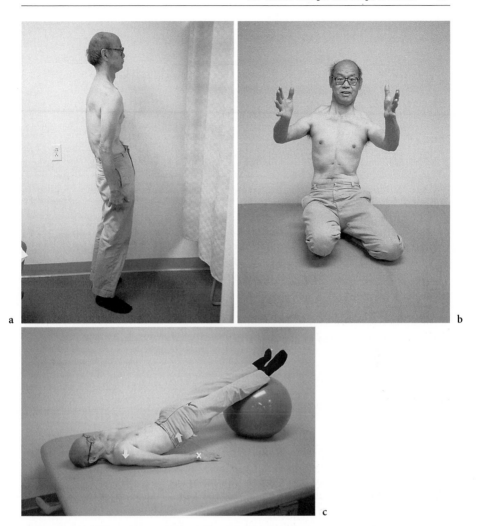

Fig 7.2 a. Posture of patient with muscular dystrophy (shoulder girdle). **b, c.** The patient is unable to raise his arms against gravity but is able to extend the hips against gravity.

Observing Range of Motion

Although it is difficult to observe ROM of hip extension while the patient is in supine position (unless the hips are lifted), this position is nevertheless *valuable for observing hip and knee flexion,* knee extension, and ankle dorsi- and plantar flexion.

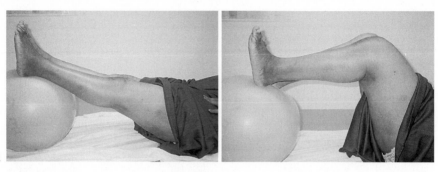

a   b

Fig. 7.3 a, b. Patient after total knee replacement; both legs demonstrate ROM of full extension and limited flexion of both knees.

EXAMPLES

Figure 7.3. A patient demonstrates her active ROM after a total knee replacement. The therapist can place the goniometer along the lower leg and thigh to measure the range without simultaneously having to hold the leg.

Dorsi- and Plantar Flexion of the Ankle

EXAMPLES

Figure 7.4. Panels a, b. A patient suffering from leukemia demonstrates how ROM of the dorsi- and plantar flexion can be assessed. The gastrocnemius muscle is not assessed here because the knee is not extended.

Panel c. Assessing hamstring muscle length and active knee extension against gravity (provided the shortness of hamstring muscles does not prevent knee extension). Shortness of the hamstring muscles and of active knee extension can be observed. In this position the gastrocnemius muscle can be assessed by adding dorsiflexion to the foot while the knee is extended.

Observing Range of Motion with Patient Sitting on a Swiss Ball. ROM of knee flexion and extension and ankle dorsi- and plantar flexion can be observed when sitting on a Swiss ball.

EXAMPLES

Figure 7.5. A child (suffering from leukemia) in intensive care demonstrates pushing and pulling the ball through the full range of the ankle movement (with flexed knees the range of the soleus muscle is tested more than the range of the gastrocnemius muscle) using the quadriceps and hamstring muscles to do so. In this very weak patient the weight of the body rests on the ball, reducing the effort required to move.

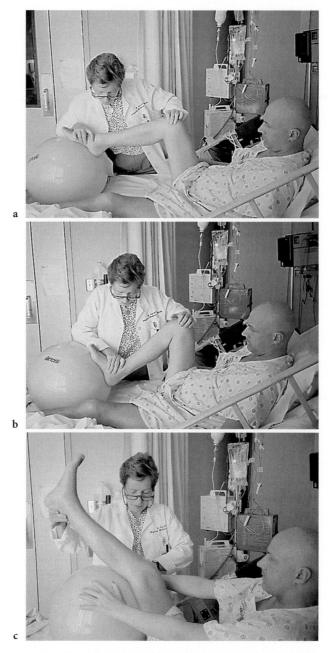

Fig. 7.4 a, b. Patient suffering from leukemia is assisted in ROM of the ankle plantar, and dorsiflexion. **c.** The patient demonstrates hamstring tightness resulting in decreased knee extension.

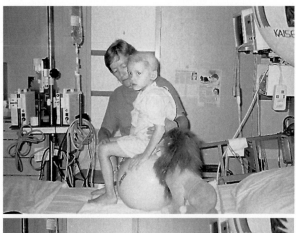

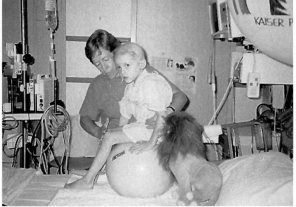

Fig. 7.5 a, b. Child with leukemia in intensive care, strengthening the quadriceps and hamstring muscles and moving the ankles through full range while the weight of the trunk is supported by the Swiss ball.

7.2.1 Hip Extensor and Flexor Muscles: Testing Strength in Side-Lying Position

> Gravity-eliminated strength of the hip extensor and flexor muscles can best be tested in a side-lying position because their axis of movement is spatially vertical. The movement takes place in a horizontal sagittal plane.

The hip abductor muscles must lift the leg (concentrically) against gravity to keep the leg in the air. Their axis of movement is spatially horizontal, and abduction of the leg takes place in a vertical frontal plane. A small Swiss ball (45 cm) placed under the upper leg when in the side-lying position enables the patient to move the leg into flexion and extension while relieving the ab-

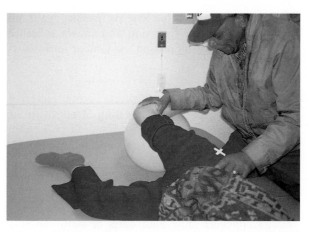

Fig. 7.6. A patient who had suffered a stroke resulting in weakness of the right side of her body is helped by her husband to move the leg into flexion and extension of the right hip.

ductors from having to lift the leg. This is important to consider when testing a patient with weakness affecting several muscles around the pelvic girdle. The test position is also used for exercise.

EXAMPLES

Figure 7.6. A patient had suffered a stroke resulting in weakness of the right side of her body is helped by her husband to move the leg while in the side-lying position into flexion and extension of the right hip.

To help in performing gravity-eliminated flexion and extension of the knee a small Swiss ball (45 cm) can be placed under the lower leg if the hip abductor muscles cannot hold the weight of the leg against gravity.

Range of Motion of the Hip

Side-Lying. The side-lying position is helpful especially in recognizing movement deficits of hip extension. If the therapist places one hand on the pelvis, as in Fig. 7.6, the movement of the pelvis can be felt instantly. With normal ROM of hip extension, the pelvis moves anteriorly/caudally only when the thigh is extended 5°–10° past neutral.

Substitution. With a shortened rectus femoris muscle, the ROM of hip extension at the hip joint decreases as the knee flexes. Substitution begins when the pelvis begins to tilt anteriorly/caudally, causing the lumbar lordosis to compensate for lack of extension.

Standing. While standing, one leg can be placed on the Swiss ball with the knee bent and the weight of the lower leg resting on the ball. In such a position the patient can practice hip extension of the leg on the ball.

Substitution. A tight rectus femoris muscle, again, prevents the hip joint from reaching neutral hip extension and causes substitution by tilting the pelvis anteriorly/caudally, increasing the lumbar lordosis.

7.2.2 Hip Extensor Muscles: Testing Strength in Supine Position

Bridging in supine position to extend the hips requires muscle activity of the hip extensor muscles against gravity. The axis of movement for flexion and extension is spatially horizontal. The sagittal plane of movement is spatially vertical. Since the legs are resting on the ball, their weight is reduced. The size of the bridge determines how difficult it is to contract the hip extensor muscles concentrically. Both heels or both calves can be placed on a Swiss ball when extending the hips and lifting the pelvis. The therapist should note

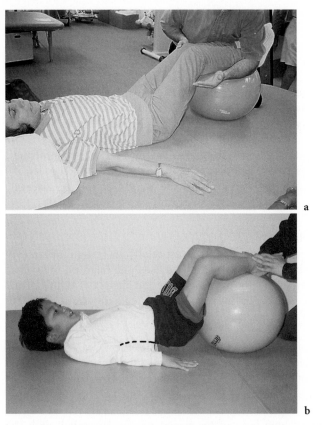

Fig. 7.7 a. A patient in the early recovery phase of transverse myelitis is unable to extend the hips against gravity. **b.** Substitution with back extension for weakness of the hip extensor muscles in a child with muscular dystrophy.

whether it is easier for the patient to lift with the smaller bridge (Swiss ball under calves) or with a larger bridge construction (Swiss ball under heels).

> **EXAMPLES**
>
> *Figure 7.7a.* A weak patient with muscle strength 1/5 or 2/5 is unable to lift her hips off the mat against gravity (a patient in the early recovery phase of transverse myelitis).

Substitution. The therapist must observe the movement sequence closely because a patient may substitute his weakness of the hip extensor muscles by using his back extensor muscles. If this substitution is taking place, the back is lifted before the hips.

> **EXAMPLES**
>
> *Figure 7.7b.* The patient arches his back to substitute for weaknesses of the hip extensor muscles instead of lifting his hips (a child with muscular dystrophy affecting the pelvic girdle).

7.2.3 Hip Extensor Muscles: Testing Strength in Prone Position

Hip extensor muscle strength can also be tested against gravity when the patient is positioned on all fours with the ball under the abdomen or while lying prone over the ball. The patient can then try to lift one leg against gravity in an open chain (free-play function). Because the axis of motion is spatially horizontal, the weight of the leg must be lifted. The sagittal plane of movement is vertical.

> **EXAMPLES**
>
> *Figure 7.8.* A patient suffering from low back problems (spondylolisthesis, old compression fracture) lifts her right leg in prone position over a Swiss ball (to protect the back). In a more acute phase the patient's muscle strength can be tested with the patient in side-lying position.
> As a progression from side-lying position, the leg can be placed on a ball while testing and exercising on the ball in prone position so that the patient can contract the muscles without having to lift the weight of the leg.
> *Figure 7.9.* A child affected by pelvic girdle muscular dystrophy (Duchenne) demonstrates his inability to extend his hips and raise the legs while prone over a PhysioRoll and a Swiss ball. Healthy persons are able to lift both legs through the full range and take resistance.

Substitution

EXAMPLES

Figure 7.9. The lack of hip extension as well as substitution for weakness of the hip abductor and external rotators muscles can be observed. The patient turns his legs inward (internal rotation of the hips); his knees are together and his feet are apart to compensate for the weakness.

Another frequent substitution for the lack of extension of the hips is extension of the head (and lumbar spine). Some patients open the mouth to facilitate extension of the head and neck.

The therapist should also observe the quality of movement: when a patient is substituting, the movement may be jerky and not in a straight line.

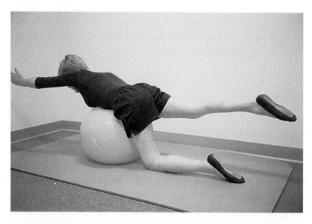

Fig. 7.8. Patient with low back problems (spondylolisthesis) lifting her right leg against gravity while protecting the back.

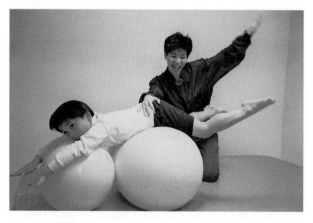

Fig. 7.9. Child with muscular dystrophy affecting the pelvic girdle is unable to extend the hips against gravity.

7.2.4   Hip Abductor and Adductor Muscles: Testing Strength in Supine Position

> The axis of movement for hip abduction and adduction *is vertical in supine and prone positions; the movement therefore carried out with gravity eliminated.* Although no weight must be lifted by the hip flexor muscles, the friction between the leg and the surface should be considered. To reduce the friction therapists can use "powder boards" or sling suspensions.

Using a Swiss ball is another way of decreasing surface friction. The Swiss ball, even a smaller one, flexes the leg slightly at the hip. In such a position the frontal plane of movement for abduction and adduction is not truly horizontal unless the therapist takes special care in positioning the patient with the feet over the edge of the mat table on a ball lower than the mat. Such an adjustment is generally not necessary, but the therapist should be aware that the movement is not taking place in a neutral hip extension.

Placing one foot on the ball decreases the strain on the hip flexor and abdominal muscles which would otherwise have to hold the leg up in the air. This use of the ball should be considered when a patient is weak or not allowed to strain the abdominal muscles, such as after abdominal surgery. Hip

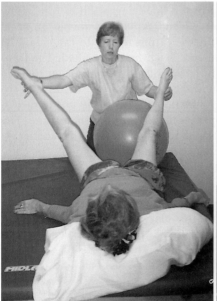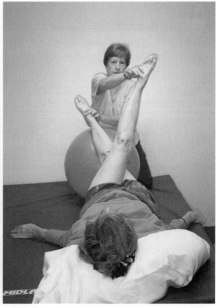

a

b

Fig. 7.10a, b. Patient with multiple sclerosis moving the left leg in an almost transverse plane into horizontal abduction and adduction. The right leg is moving in an almost frontal plane into abduction and adduction with the right hip almost extended.

abduction and adduction can also be done in a transverse plane of movement (horizontal abduction and adduction). This requires well-stretched hamstrings and good muscle strength (at least 3/5) because the weight of the leg must be held and then moved at 90° hip flexion in an open kinetic chain.

EXAMPLES

Figure 7.10. A patient with the diagnosis of *multiple sclerosis* is assisted by the therapist. The patient's right leg is much weaker than the left leg and can be moved into abduction and adduction only while resting on the ball. This exercise is adapted from the "Pendulum" exercise (see Sect. 9.23; Klein-Vogelbach 1990b,c; Carrière 1993).

Range of Motion. One can evaluate ROM either when the patient is moving the leg actively, or when the therapist is moving the leg passively into hip abduction and adduction while it is positioned on the Swiss ball. To prevent the leg from "falling" off the ball during abduction of the hip the leg can be placed off center at the beginning of the movements so that it is still on the ball when the leg is abducted.

7.2.5 Hip Abductor and Adductor Muscles: Testing Strength in Side-Lying Position

Strength against gravity of the hip abductor muscles (and lateral trunk muscles) in a bridge activity are best tested in the side-lying position (preferably over a PhysioRoll for stability). If a Swiss ball is used, a wedge or towel should be placed alongside to prevent the ball from rolling to the side. The axis of movement is spatially horizontal and weight must be lifted. The frontal plane of movement is spatially vertical. Both legs are resting on the ball in the side-lying position on the ball, and the pelvis is lifted. To test the abductor muscles of the hip in free-play function the trunk is positioned in side-lying on a PhysioRoll, and the upper leg is lifted in a frontal plane. The lever of the leg can be short (bent leg) or long (extended leg), depending on the weight of the leg and the strength of the patient. The patient can compare sides to determine which is weaker and needs strengthening.

EXAMPLES

Figure 7.11. The patient has at least a muscle strength of 3/5 or more to be able to lift the upper leg in a free-play function (and the trunk into lateral flexion). The hip abductor muscles of the lower leg are activated in a bridge activity.

The leg can also be placed in abduction on the Swiss ball, and the patient can then try to lift the leg off the ball.

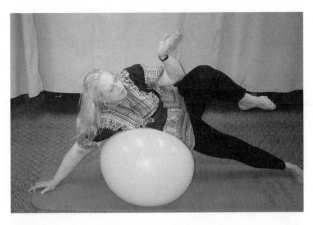

Fig. 7.11. Patient lifting her left leg with shortened lever into abduction in an open kinetic chain. The right leg is in a bridge activity.

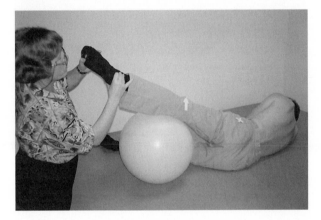

Fig. 7.12. Patient substituting abduction by externally rotating left leg while trying to lift the leg.

Substitution

EXAMPLES

Figure 7.12. If the patient is unable to abduct the leg, he may substitute by externally rotating the leg to recruit his hip flexor muscles to lift the leg.

7.2.6 Combination of Movements in Several Planes

Normal strength (and coordination) is required in the more difficult version of the "Pendulum" exercise. The hips are extended in a bridge activity and

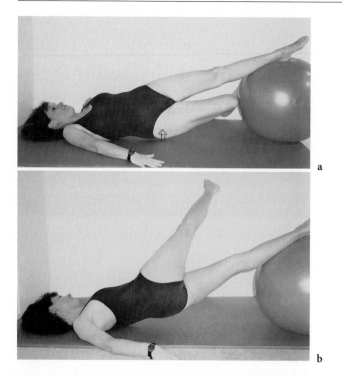

Fig. 7.13 a. Rotating the pelvic girdle, the left hip adductor muscles are activated in a bridge activity (closed chain); the right hip adductor muscles are activated in an open kinetic chain. **b.** Right hip abductor muscles in an open chain, left hip abductor muscles in a bridge activity.

then rotated (Fig. 7.13a). In the first position the hip adductor muscles of the upper leg are in a bridge activity, while the hip adductor muscles of the lower leg are activated in a free-play function holding the weight of the leg. During the next phase the abductor muscles of the lower leg are activated in a bridge activity, while abductor muscles of the upper leg hold the weight of the leg in a free-play function (Fig. 7.13b). This very challenging exercise activates the entire rotator "cuff" of the hip joint and combines testing for strength, skill, and coordination.

7.3 Back Extensor and Trapezius Muscles: Testing Strength

Patients with weaknesses of the middle back cannot lift the upper extremities in the sagittal (forward flexion), frontal (abduction), or transverse plane (horizontal abduction) of movement when positioned prone over a Swiss ball.

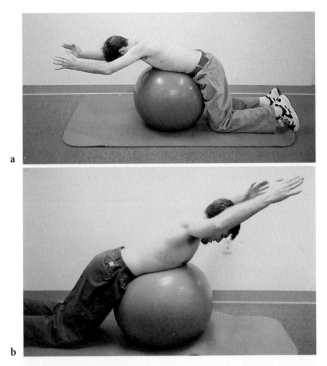

Fig. 7.14 a. Patient demonstrating weakness of the back extensor muscles and the trapezius muscle approximately 3 weeks after a motor vehicle accident. **b.** Approximately 4 months later, his muscle strength is normal.

EXAMPLES

Figure 7.14. Panel a. The patient was seen 3 weeks after a motor vehicle accident which resulted in internal injuries and required abdominal surgery. In the recovery phase the patient suffered from weight loss and general weakness.

Resting in prone position over the Swiss ball with approximately 80° hip flexion, the patient was unable to actively extend the back. Weakness of the lower trapezius and back extensor muscles was apparent (approximately grade 3–/5) while observing his inability to lift the arms against gravity in elongation of the trunk.

Panel b. Four months later, after following a home exercise program, the patient's strength had returned to normal (5/5) for the trunk extensor muscles and lower trapezius muscle.

Figure 7.15. Panel a. The patient (same as in Fig. 7.2) exhibits profound weakness when lifting his arms in the sagittal plane against gravity. The axes of movement for flexion and extension of the arms and the trunk are horizontal in space.

Panel b. With the weight of the arm resting on the Swiss ball, the patient is able to reduce the amount of weight of the arm on the ball,

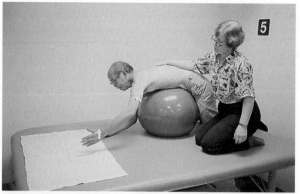

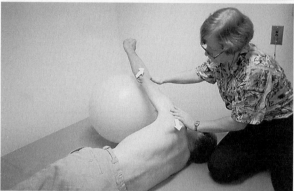

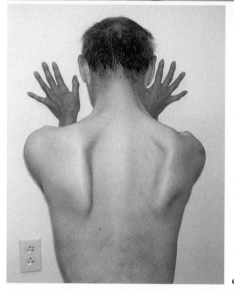

Fig. 7.15 a–e. Patient with muscular dystrophy. **a.** Inability to lift upper extremities in a vertical sagittal plane against gravity. **b.** Inability to lift arm off the Swiss ball in a transverse plane but the patient is able to contract muscles. **c.** Weakness of the serratus and rhomboid muscles. **d.** Inability to contact shoulder girdle muscles in a horizontal transverse plane of movement. **e.** Inability to raise shoulders in a frontal plane, activating upper trapezius muscles with weight of arms supported on Swiss ball.

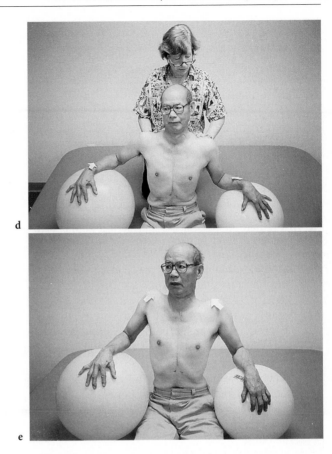

Fig. 7.15 d, e

d

e

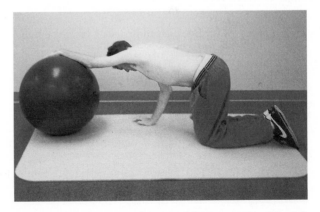

Fig. 7.16. Patient with kyphotic posture and decreased ROM of back extension. The left shoulder is elevated.

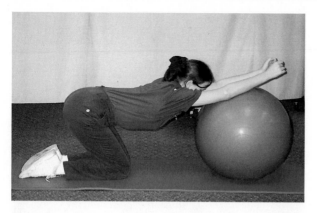

Fig. 7.17. Healthy person demonstrating normal ROM of back extension.

but he is unable to lift the arm in the transverse plane of the body into horizontal abduction.

Panel c. The *rhomboid, serratus, and deltoid muscles* are also very weak.

Panel d. The patient is able to contract the muscles by pulling the shoulder blades together if the weight of the arms is resting on two Swiss balls.

Panel e. The patient is using the same starting position to raise his shoulders and activate the upper *trapezius muscles* through part of the range in a vertical frontal plane of movement. The patient can do so without substitution because the weight of the arms is resting on the balls.

Substitution

EXAMPLES

Figure 7.15a. Because the patient lacked extension of the trunk he extended his head.

Range of Motion

EXAMPLES

Figure 7.16. The patient demonstrates poor mobility of trunk extension.

Figure 7.17. The person demonstrates normal ROM of trunk extension and shoulder forward flexion.

7.4 Triceps Brachii Muscle: Testing Strength

The triceps brachii muscle can be tested for good or normal strength by positioning the patient prone over the ball with the hands on the floor.

> It is important to watch the position of hands and elbows.

The hands should point forward while the elbows should be slightly bent and pointing toward the abdomen and not to the sides. The shoulders should be positioned over the hands; for stronger muscles they can be spatially in front of the hands while performing a push-up (Fig. 5.1). Very good strength is required because the axis of movement is spatially horizontal and part of the body weight hangs on the triceps. The sagittal plane of movement is spatially vertical. When a patient is sitting and resting the forearm on a Swiss ball, the triceps brachii muscle can be tested gravity-eliminated by moving the Swiss ball to extend the elbow.

Substitution

> **EXAMPLES**
>
> *Figure 5.1b.* The load on the triceps brachii muscle decreases if the elbows are turned outward during the push-up; the shoulders are not over the hands, and the ball is moving more cranially during the exercise.

7.5 Abdominal Muscles and Hip Flexor Muscles (Iliopsoas): Testing Strength in Sitting Position

Normal muscle strength of the abdominal and the iliopsoas muscles is demonstrated in Fig. 5.3 a. by a healthy subject performing the "Scale" exercise (see Sect. 9.2), which can also be done with the arms elevated increasing the demand on the abdominal muscles. When the patient has a long trunk and short leg and/or a comparatively large head or a heavy shoulder girdle (e.g., muscle bulk in patients who lift weights), the "Scale" exercise is more difficult.

A patient with weak abdominal muscles should rest the weight of the arms on the lap and reduce the amount of backward leaning (requiring eccentric muscle activity).

Figure 7.19. Panel a. The patient demonstrates his weakness and lack of awareness of the alignment. Unable to stand up without help, he compensates for his weakness with a wide BOS and by pushing his knees together to stabilize himself.

Panel b. The patient tries to align his legs but keeps the right knee in slight valgus position.

Possible causes of poor alignment include:

- Poor habit and the lack of awareness of the position of the leg or legs
- Weakness, especially of the vastus medialis of the quadriceps femoris muscle
- Tightness of muscles such as hamstring muscles, tensor fascia latae, or hip flexor muscles
- Substitution for lack of pronation of the forefoot
- Eversion of the calcaneus
- Increased muscle tonus on the lower extremities
- Decreased balance
- Altered proprioception, for example, after surgery, injury
- Medical conditions such as degenerative arthritis of hip or knee joints or after surgeries, and fractures

The Swiss ball can be used to evaluate the ability to align the legs, and it may help to identify the cause of the misalignment. Muscle tightness of the

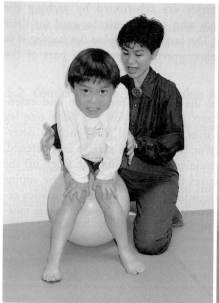
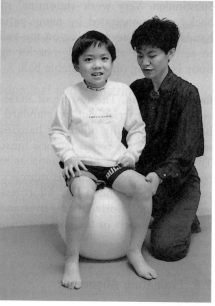

a
b

Fig. 7.19 a. Patient demonstrating lack of awareness of the lower extremity alignment. **b.** The patient cannot stand up unassisted.

lower extremities (especially hamstring muscles and tensor fascia latae) combined with decreased ROM (especially lack of pronation of the forefoot) is common in patients with problems of their feet such as: painful heel spurs, hallux valgus, and plantar fascitis. Patients with patella-femoral complaints usually also have alignment problems. Patients should be able to move the well-aligned leg at normal gait velocity (Inman 1982; Whittle 1991; Perry 1992; Bronner 1992; Carrière 1993; Wu 1994; Klein-Vogelbach 1995) without having to concentrate on the task.

EXAMPLES

Figure 7.20. The patient suffered from severe pain in her feet after several hallux valgus surgeries.
- The left leg had greater alignment problems than the right leg (Fig. 7.20a). The patient was evaluated for her alignment and able to correct the faulty movement pattern when:
- Sitting on a stable surface (Fig. 7.20b)
- Moving the leg positioned on a ball while sitting on a stable surface (Fig. 7.20c)
- Lying in supine position with the feet placed on the ball
- Sitting on the ball, moving forward/back and hopping (Fig. 7.20d)
- Bicycling
- Walking on a treadmill

At first the patient was unable to correct her alignment without external cues and could not move the legs correctly at normal gait velocity. The patient worked diligently at home to correct the faulty alignment, to mobilize the forefoot into pronation, and to strengthen her lower extremity muscles. She became free of pain after a few sessions of instructions and reevaluation of alignment.

Making the patient aware of the problem enables him to correct it.

Dots can be used to increase awareness and to observe the alignment. Coins can be taped onto the floor under the outside of the heel and under the base of the big toe to give tactile feedback. A mirror can be placed in front of the patient for visual feedback when evaluating alignment. The patient can then correct the problem. At a later stage of recovery the patient should not require any cues as the alignment should be automatic.

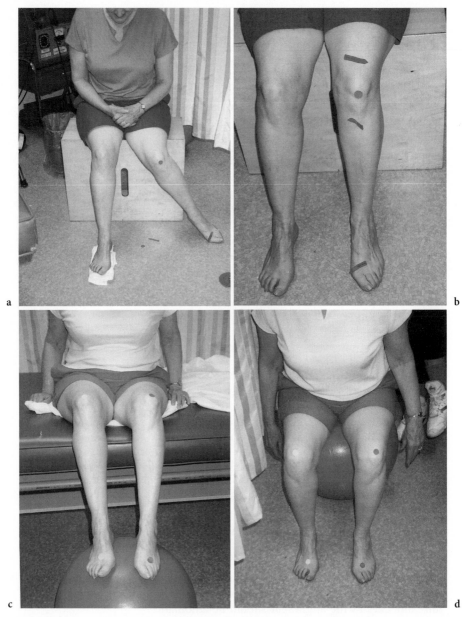

Fig. 7.20 a. Patient demonstrating her faulty alignment, left leg more than right leg. **b.** Correcting the alignment while sitting on a stable surface. **c.** Patient sitting on a stable surface correcting the alignment while moving the leg positioned on a ball. **d.** Correcting alignment while sitting on the ball, moving forward/back and hopping.

Fig. 7.21. Therapist is assisting the patient to move her left paralyzed leg after a stroke.

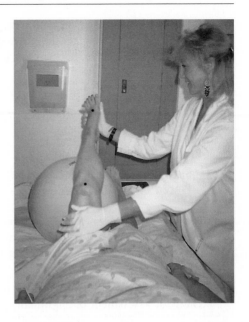

7.6.1 Supine Position with the Swiss Ball Under One Leg

From the beginning the therapist should move a weak or paralyzed leg in proper alignment and try to teach the patient to do so when he can move the leg himself.

EXAMPLES

Figure 7.21. The patient who had a stroke causing weakness on the left side of the body observes the leg and the dots during passive movement.

7.6.2 Common Patterns of Deviation from Normal Alignment of Femur, Lower Leg, and Foot

- A patient recovering from a stroke tends to move the paralyzed leg into abduction and external rotation of the hip.
- A patient with spasticity may pull his leg into flexion and adduction at the hip joints.
- A patient with decreased proprioception and instability has difficulty moving the leg in a straight line.
- A patient with mild weakness and tightness of some muscles of the lower extremity must concentrate and observe the movement to execute it correctly.

- A patient with decreased pronation of the forefoot is able to align the leg only when concentrating on the movement and when positioned in supine position with the calf or heel on the ball because the forefoot is not fixed in pronation.

Changing faulty movement patterns takes time. The habit of substituting persists and affects the alignment until the correct pattern becomes automatic.

7.6.3 Sitting on a Bench/Chair and with the Swiss Ball Placed Under the Feet

One or both feet can be placed on the ball while moving it in a straight line. The BOS is mobile and decreased. It may be more difficult for patients to keep the knee well aligned while moving the foot forward and back.

> Patients who lack balance for sitting on the Swiss ball can sit on a chair for assessment of alignment.

7.6.4 Sitting on the Swiss Ball

The same problems as those described above can be observed when sitting on a ball (and moving back and forth) or hopping. However, it is more difficult for the patient to correct the problem because the feet are on the ground and balance becomes an issue. Neurological deficits become more apparent.

> Patients with decreased pronation of the forefoot may be able to align the foot and the knee only by lifting the first metatarsal/phalanx off the floor. This can be observed frequently in patients with foot problems such as hallux valgus, plantar fascitis, pes planus, etc.

Joint or soft tissue mobilization may be required to mobilize the forefoot into pronation.

7.6.5 Sitting on the Swiss Ball and Taking Steps Until Reaching Supine Position on the Swiss Ball

Alignment and balance can be evaluated while sitting on a Swiss ball and taking steps. Steps can be taken on the spot, or the patient can take steps forward until positioned in supine on the ball.

Fig. 7.22. Patient suffering from multiple sclerosis requires help from the therapist secondary to weakness and alignment problems and proprioceptive/balance deficits.

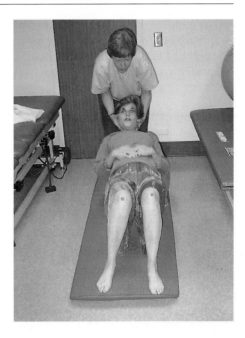

<table>
<tr><td>EXAMPLES</td><td>*Figure 7.22.* Moving from a sitting to a supine position, a patient suffering from multiple sclerosis needs help from the therapist to reach the end position. The lack of alignment in the right leg is due to weakness, decreased proprioception, and impaired balance.</td></tr>
</table>

7.7 Evaluating Quality of Movement and Dissociation of the Lower Extremities

A patient walked into our physical therapy department 4 months after having sustained a head trauma in a motor vehicle accident. He also had a fracture of the femur of his right leg; the therapist noticed that the patient had some problems walking, but he did not use a cane. It was difficult to pinpoint his problem, although it was noticeable that the right side of his body lacked harmony of movement. After taking the history the therapist tested strength and alignment with the Swiss ball. Problem areas were assessed by manual muscle testing. Muscle tonus and quality of movement were evaluated simultaneously with the Swiss ball. This helped the therapist to determine whether both sides of the body were affected and to what extent. The patient was first tested in the most stable position: supine. This also enabled the patient safely to become accustomed to the challenge of the Swiss ball.

The following skills can be evaluated in addition to strength:
- Quality of movement of one leg or both legs
- Ability to dissociate leg
- Problems arising from movement at gait velocity

7.7.1 Supine Position, Both Legs on the Swiss Ball

The patient rests on his back, and both legs are placed with the calves on a small or medium-sized Swiss ball (45 or 55 cm diameter). He is asked to move both legs into flexion and extension of hips and knees while the therapist assesses the direction, speed, and quality of movement. When the legs extend, the therapist can observe the knees to determine whether one leg hyperextends more than the other (which may indicate poor eccentric control of the hamstring muscles).

The therapist may also let the patient resist lateral movements while gently pushing the ball to compare stability of each side of the trunk, both with the pelvis on the mat and with the pelvis lifted.

> The therapist should also observe the patient's arms. Do they rest on the mat next to the hips? Are they positioned symmetrical? Does the patient have difficulty keeping one arm down, indicating associated reactions and/or changes of muscle tonus?

7.7.2 Supine Position, One Leg Resting on the Swiss Ball

Still in the supine position, the patient is asked to move one leg at a time into flexion and extension, and the quality of movement can be compared with that in the other leg. The exercise is more difficult when only the heel is positioned on the ball, especially if the patient has long legs.

7.7.3 Supine Position with Alternate Leg Movements

One Leg on the Swiss Ball, Pelvis on the Mat

The patient is asked to move the legs alternately as in the exercise "Perpetual Motion" (see Sect. 9.22; Klein-Vogelbach 1990b,c; Carrière 1993). It is easier to keep the more involved leg on the ball while flexing and extending the other one in the air. Again, the therapist observes the quality of movement.

> Can the patient move the leg on the ball smoothly into flexion while the other leg is extending into the air? Can the patient keep the other leg flexed while extending the leg on the ball? Can the legs perform the movements in a straight line, smoothly and with increased speed?

One Leg on the Swiss ball, Pelvis Lifted

In this position (see Sect. 9.22, exercise "Perpetual Motion"), the therapist can observe and compare sides if the patient is able to:

- Lift his pelvis and keep one leg extended with the heel (or calf) on the ball and flex the other leg in the air.
- Keep the trunk and arms stable while moving the legs and lifting the pelvis each time that one leg is extended and the other flexed.

The therapist may discover that the patient has weakness in addition to difficulty in performing the exercise, even when it was demonstrated or the patient was well instructed. The patient may demonstrate difficulty coordinating the movements of the legs and lack truck stability even on the presumably "uninvolved" side.

7.7.4 Prone Position Over the Swiss Ball

The patient can also be tested in prone over the ball. The exercises "Salamander," "Swing," or "Crab" (Sects. 9.9, 9.10, 9.12; Klein-Vogelbach 1990b, 1991; Carrière 1993) may help the therapist to observe the coordination of hands and feet while the trunk is supported on the Swiss ball, preferably a ball with a diameter of 55 cm or more, depending on the length of the trunk and extremities. The patient should fit comfortably over the ball.

If the patient does well in the supine or prone position, the therapist can test both coordination and balance as the patient sits on the Swiss ball.

7.8 Testing Balance

7.8.1 Balance Deficits

> Good balance requires postural control (strength and mobility), intact vision, hearing, and proprioception. Alertness, attention, and memory may also be important to avoid loss of balance.

If a person remembers that there is a hole around the sprinkler and pays attention while walking across the lawn, he is less likely to fall or lose his balance when stepping into the hole. The following example demonstrates the importance of vision and proprioception.

EXAMPLES A patient who had suffered a stroke and was able to ambulate well with a cane on level surfaces went on a cruise. She enjoyed the trip and did well until a storm rocked the boat and large waves could be seen outside the window. The patient could no longer rely on her vision, vestibular equilibrium, or proprioception since the world around her was moving. "I became unable to walk. I thought I had another stroke," the patient said, "I had to stay in bed until the storm was over; then I could walk again, and I realized that I was all right."

Falling and loss of balance has been well studied in older adults (Duncan et al. 1993a; Lord et al. 1991; Tinetti and Ginter 1988; Duncan et al. 1992; Gehlsen and Whaley 1990; Weiner et al. 1992) and has been attributed to decreased strength and mobility as well as to somatosensory/sensorimotor, visual and vestibular problems. Balance cannot be reflected by any single measure but is instead multifactorial; balance problems reflect an accumulation of deficits across several domains (Duncan et al. 1993b).

Studies of the effect of exercise on balance strength and reaction time in the elderly have found significant improvements in strength and body sway following an exercise program compared to those who do not exercise (Lord and Castell 1994).

Sensorimotor receptors are located in the skin, joints, tendons, ligaments and muscles (Allison 1995). Neurological injuries such as multiple sclerosis, Guillain-Barré syndrome, spinal cord injury, and peripheral neuropathy can cause *damage to the sensorimotor system*. Orthopedic and surgical injuries such as fractures, sprains, and amputation can also *affect proprioception and sensation*. Peripheral *visual loss and decreased sensation* can occur in patients with diabetes. Cataracts and glaucoma may *impair the vision* of older patients. Menière's disease and acoustic neuroma may *influence the peripheral vestibular system* and cause balance problems.

Central sensory perception plays an important role in comparing the inputs between the two sides of the body and the three primary sensory systems (Allison 1995).

The inability to integrate visual, vestibular, and somatosensory information for midline orientation is illustrated by Allison (1995) in the case of a hemiplegic patient with "pusher syndrome." Gill-Body et al. (1994) present two case reports on peripheral vestibular dysfunction.

Central motor planning (see also Chap. 2) prepares and affects movements as well, including the ability to scale movements and subconsciously to adjust muscles when reaching, for example, for an empty or a full glass of water. The skill improves with training. A healthy person usually knows whether the surface that he is planning to sit on is mobile or stable, and automatically adjusts his muscles accordingly. Reflexes (such as vestibulo-ocular and vestibulo-spinal) and righting reactions are seen early in child development (Allison 1995).

> Automatic postural responses assist in keeping the center of gravity over the BOS. In addition, anticipatory postural responses and volitional postural movements are also involved in maintaining balance. Numerous tests have been recommended for assessment of balance impairments (e.g., Allison's chapter 1995; see also the various other works mentioned above), all of which are very valuable. Some begin the testing in standing position and others in gait. Some patients cannot walk but still need to work on balance. Training the patient's sitting balance may prepare him for standing and walking. The problem is that most therapists cannot perform the recommended tests because of limited time and space.

Risk factors for older adults to be fallers include muscle weakness, poor balance, gait abnormalities, and slow response time (MacRae et al. 1992). All these risk facors can be addressed with Swiss ball exercises.

7.8.2 Screening Balance

The Swiss ball can be used to screen and evaluate balance problems since "having a client sitting on a gymnastic ball doing almost any exercise will require vestibular and proprioceptive feedback to make the appropriate adaptive responses" (Umphred 1995). In addition, it is a valuable tool in working on postural control and strength.

Biesinger et al. (1991) describe a functional treatment progression for peripheral and central balance deficits. The following sequence of Swiss ball exercises may be useful for patients who are suspected of having primary central/postural balance deficits, both for evaluation/screening and for treatment. The patient obtains feedback about his performance and can practice at home. This is important because only a few patients have the luxury of frequent treatments in a physical therapy practice. Success is "measurable" because the exercises can be adapted to the patient's ability and can be made more difficult as the patient becomes more skilled.

> To enhance learning the patient should begin with exercises that he can perform and progress to more difficult exercises rather than to begin practicing those that he is unable to do.

The suggested progression is:
1. Supine position
2. Sitting on a stable surface

3. Sitting on a Swiss ball (unstable surface)
4. Sitting on a Swiss ball and placing the feet on an unstable surface
5. Hopping on a Swiss ball
6. Kneeling on an unstable surface, holding on to a Swiss ball
7. Standing on an unstable surface

Supine Position

EXAMPLES

Figure 7.2c. When a patient is bridging with his calves or feet on the ball, there may be an instant movement of the ball to one side if the trunk control is insufficient.

In other patients, a difference in stability on each side of the trunk becomes apparent when giving resistance to the ball which the patient is attempting to keep stable. The therapist can cue the patient at first by briefly touching the leg on the side that the patient must activate for the resistance.

Sitting on a Stable Surface. Before sitting the patient on the ball it may be beneficial to evaluate static and dynamic balance on a stable surface. With the patient sitting on a chair or mat table, the therapist can evaluate static and dynamic trunk control by observing whether the patient is able to sit unsupported and then challenge the balance by gently pushing the patient.

Sitting on an Unstable Surface (Swiss Ball). The patient can sit on the Swiss ball with a wide base (feet placed apart). External support can be provided by the therapist holding onto the patient's trunk, or the patient holding onto two chairs placed alongside, in between parallel bars, or holding onto a mat table. The patient can then balance himself with the arms stretched out at the sides and keeping a wide triangular BOS.

EXAMPLES

Figure 7.23. The hands can join and the BOS be decreased while sitting on the Swiss ball. The physical therapist can give minimal external support (if needed) and verbal feedback or challenge the balance.

The patient can progress to performing the exercise with eyes closed. The therapist must guard against possible loss of balance and swaying to one or both sides. As a progression, these exercises can also be done sitting on a balance board.

Fig. 7.23. The hands can be joined for stabilization, and the BOS decreased while sitting on the Swiss ball.

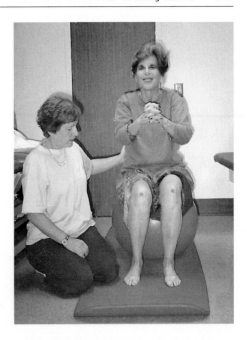

Sitting on a Swiss Ball with an Unstable Surface Under the Feet

EXAMPLES

Figure 7.24. Panel a. An unstable surface is placed under the feet while the patient is sitting on the Swiss ball.

Panel b. In the beginning an alternative for sitting on the Swiss ball is to let the patient sit on the Sitfit and place the feet on another Sitfit. The therapist can also use a piece of foam, a foam roll, a small tilt board, or the Sitfit which is almost like a flat ball, and as a progression, sit on a firm ball and place the feet on a Sitfit or other unstable surface.

Figure 7.25. A patient suffering from poliomyelitis in his right lower leg (the right foot is 2 sizes smaller than the left foot) balances while sitting on the Swiss ball, with eyes closed and the right foot planted on a stable surface. The patient was unable to perform the same exercise with the right foot on an unstable surface.

Panels a–c. He balances himself only when the left foot bears weight on the Sitfit.

Panel d. Five weeks later, after having practiced the skill at home, the patient is able to balance with eyes closed and only his right lower leg positioned on a Sitfit.

Figure 7.26. For greater challenge in patients able to function at a higher level (e.g., ambulating without a cane) two Sitfits can be placed under the feet. The patient is then asked to fix his gaze while performing the exercises on the Swiss ball to train movements affecting the vestibulo-ocular reflexes.

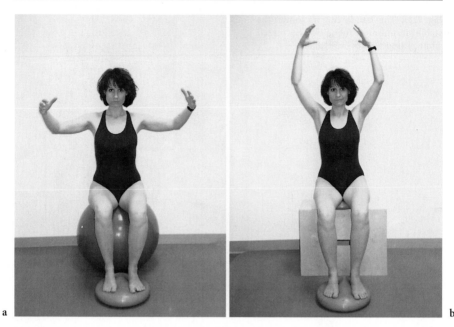

Fig. 7.24 a. Demonstration of sitting on the Swiss ball with a Sitfit under the feet. **b.** An alternative is to sit on a Sitfit and to have the feet on another Sitfit.

Hopping on the Swiss Ball. The patient can hop with erect posture while sitting on the Swiss ball, with a large or a small BOS, pushing off with both feet at the same time or alternately. If the patient does not keep contact with the Swiss ball while hopping, caution must be taken to prevent the ball from rolling away (e.g. use a Stabilizer). The patient can hop in a circle around the Swiss ball in either direction, stepping sideways or hopping. The patient can sit on the Swiss ball and try to catch a small ball.

Kneeling on a Stable/Unstable Surface

> **EXAMPLES**
>
> *Figure 7.27.* Panel a. Kneeling on a stable surface, holding onto a Swiss ball, and kneeling on one or two Sitfits requires dynamic stability. The task is more difficult if the kneeling patient has only an unstable object to hold onto, such as a Swiss ball.
> Panel b. The patient kneels on two Sitfits and balances the trunk with no support from toes or hands.

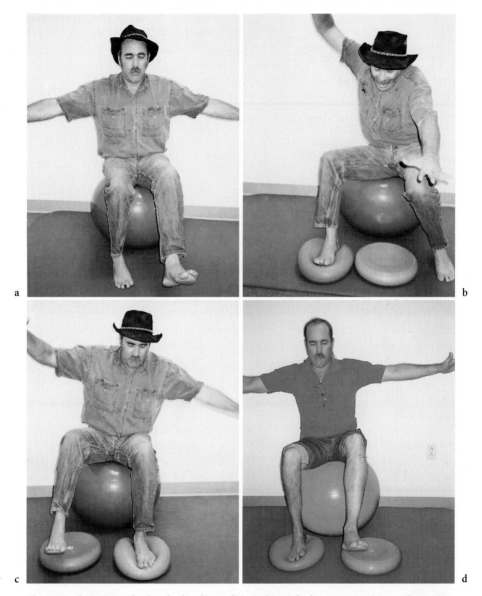

a

b

c

d

Fig. 7.25a–d. Patient who has had poliomyelitis in his right lower extremity. **a.** The patient is able to balance sitting on the Swiss ball with closed eyes, right foot planted on the mat. **b.** Inability to balance with closed eyes and right leg on unstable surface. **c.** Patient succeeds with left leg on unstable surface (Sitfit). **d.** After exercising at home the patient succeeds in balancing with the right foot on the Sitfit with eyes closed.

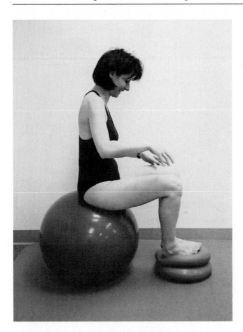

Fig. 7.26. For higher level patients having two Sitfits under the feet poses a great challenge.

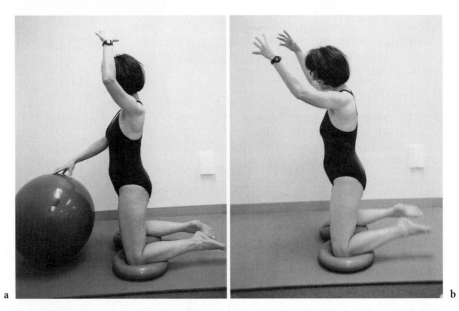

a   b

Fig. 7.27 a. Kneeling on two Sitfits holding onto a Swiss ball (unstable surface). **b.** Without support.

Fig. 7.28. Standing on two Sitfits lifting a Swiss ball.

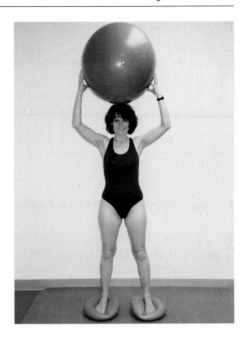

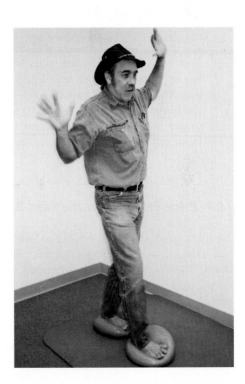

Fig. 7.29. Tandem standing on two Sitfits with open eyes. The patient was able to catch a Swiss ball.

Standing on One or Two Sitfits and Using the Swiss Ball

> *Figure 7.28.* Standing on two Sitfits demands good balance, especially if a Swiss ball is held above the head or is being thrown and caught. *Figure 7.29.* Tandem standing on two Sitfits with open or closed eyes demands great balance but can be practiced at home in a door frame or near a wall (preferably a corner) when learning the skill. The patient can then try to catch a Swiss ball.

7.9 Identifying Neurotension Problems and Treatment

It is very important to recognize neurotension problems and to integrate mobilization of the nervous system into the treatment (e.g., Butler 1991). Davies (1994) integrated concepts of nervous system mobilization into the treatment of patients with head trauma and stroke in the early recovery phase. The *slump test* for evaluating involvement of the nervous system in patients with back pain was presented by Maitland in 1986. Two years later Kenneally et al. (1988) described the *upper limb tension test* (ULTT) as the straight leg raise test of the upper extremity, and the following year Butler and Gifford (1989) developed the concept of *adverse mechanical tension* in the nervous system. Halle (1996) uses the ULTT as part of the "scan" evaluation of the thoracic spine.

> The Swiss ball is not the most ideal tool for evaluating neurotension but is valuable for the mobilization of tight neural structures. Therapists should be able to recognize when a more thorough evaluation of the nervous system is required, and when signs of referred pain are present which may be radicular or stem from other sources, such as joint, capsule, tendon, muscle, ligament, and bursa (Cyriax 1982).

7.9.1 Prone Position over the Swiss Ball

A patient positioned prone over the Swiss ball with his hand resting on the floor can have his arms in approximately 90° forward flexion in a closed kinetic chain. The fingers are often extended on the floor (unless the hand is positioned on a roll, see Sect. 8.2). If the patient has tightness in the nervous system of the upper limbs, he may not want to extend the elbows, complaining of increased tension in his forearms and or numbness/tingling in his hands. The therapist must evaluate these findings, compare the two sides and decide whether the exercise should be abandoned or adapted. Sometimes the exercise can help to mobilize the tight structures (see Figs. 2.11a,c, 2.12b).

Figure 2.12. The patient suffered from referred pain 6 months after a lumbar surgery. The Swiss ball and the PhysioRoll were used to mobilize the thoracic spine, soft tissue, and nervous structures. The position of the therapist's hands (panel b) indicate the way in which soft tissue can be mobilized. The therapist may also apply distraction (with the hand placed directly on the skin of the patient) with or without rotation into opposite directions of the hands.

Figure 7.14. The patient mobilizes his abdominal structures and the spine into extension in an open kinetic chain.

Figure 7.17. The arms are supported while the spine is mobilized into extension.

Figure 7.8. Mobilization of extension from the tip of the right toe to the tip of the left hand occurred in prone position.

Figures 2.6, 7.11 c. Lateral flexion (side bending) of the trunk was mobilized.

Figures 2.6, 8.20. Arrows indicate the placement and directions for soft tissue mobilization.

Figure 2.11c. Rotation and extension of the spine are combined.

7.9.2 Supine Position over the Swiss Ball

Supine over the Swiss ball is another position that is useful for stretching tight structures of the nervous system and the soft tissue.

Figure 4.1b. The entire ventral chain is stretched.

Figure 4.4. Some adaptations, such as pillows, limit the extension of the spine. The rectus femoris muscle is stretched because the knees are in 90° and the hips extended.

Figure 6.4b. Because of the bridge construction and the feet on the tip of the toes more mobilization into extension of the spine is taking place. The head is flexed.

Figure 6.5. With the hips flexed, the stretching occurs predominantly in the upper thoracic spine and shoulder/arms, mobilizing also soft tissue structures.

7.9.3 Supine with the Legs on the Swiss Ball

Figure 7.4c. Gentle stretching of the dorsal chain is demonstrated by letting the ball support the thigh and extending the knee. Holding the Swiss ball with the hands and lifting the head adds to the mobilization of the spine into flexion. Adding dorsiflexion to the foot would increase the mobilization of the neural structures.

Figure 7.13. Rotation of the spine is added to the extension of the spine.

There are numerous other Swiss ball exercises elsewhere in this book that are useful for mobilizating the nervous system. Many standard exercises can be modified accordingly.

References

Allison L (1995) Balance disorders. In: Umphred DA (ed) Neurological rehabilitation, 3rd edn. Mosby, St. Louis, pp 802–837

Biesinger E, Zimmermann R, Issing P, Scheinpflug B (1991) Krankengymnastisches Trainingsprogramm gegen Schwindel. Krankengymnastik 43:791–801

Bobath B (1978) Evaluation and treatment, 2nd edn. Heinemann, London

Bronner O (1992) Die untere Extremität. Pflaum, München

Butler DS (1991) Mobilisation of the nervous system. Churchill Livingston, New York

Butler DS, Gifford LS (1989) The concept of adverse mechanical tension in the nervous system. I. Testing for dural tension. Physiotherapy 75:622–629

Carrière B (1993) Swiss ball exercises. PT Magazine Phys Ther 9:92–100

Clarkson HM, Gilewich GB (1989) Musculoskeletal assessment joint range of motion and manual muscle strength. Williams & Wilkins, Baltimore

Cyriax J (1982) Textbook of orthopaedic medicine, 8th edn. Baillière Tindall & Cassell, London

Daniels L, Worthingham (1986) Muscle testing, 5th edn. Saunders, Philadelphia

Davies PM (1994) Starting again. Springer, Berlin Heidelberg New York

Duncan PW, Studenski SA, Chandler J, Prescott B (1992) Functional reach: predictive validity in a sample of elderly male veterans. J Gerontol Med Sci 47:M93–98

Duncan PW, Chandler J, Studenski S, Hughes M (1993a) How do physiological components of balance affect mobility in elderly men? Arch Phys Med Rehabil 74:1343–1349

Duncan PW, Shumway-Cook A, Whipple RH, Wolf S, Woollacott M (1993b) Is there one simple measure for balance? PT Magazine Phys Ther 1:74–81

Florence JM, Pandya S, King WM et al (1992) Intrarater reliability of manual muscle test (Medical Research Council scale) grades in Duchenne's muscular dystrophy. Phys Ther 72:115–126

Flynn TW (ed) (1996) The thoracic spine and rib case. Butterworth-Heinemann, Boston

Gehlsen G, Whaley MH (1990) Falls in the elderly: balance, strength, and flexibility. Arch Phys Med Rehabil 71:739–741

Gill-Body KM, Drebs DE, Parker SW, Riley PO (1994) Physical therapy management of peripheral vestibular dysfunction: two clinical case reports. Phys Ther 74:129–142

Halle JS (1996) Neuromusculoskeletal scan examination with selected related topics. In: Flynn TW (ed) The thoracic spine and ribcage. Butterworth-Heinemann, Boston, pp 121–146

Inman VT, Ralstone HJ, Todd F (1984) Human walking. Williams & Wilkins Baltimore, pp 22–62

Janda V (1991) Muscle spasm – a proposed procedure for differential diagnosis. J Manual Med 6:136–139

Janda V (1994a) Manuelle Muskelfunktionsdiagnostik, 3rd edn. Ullstein Mosby, Berlin

Janda V (1994b) Assessment of abnormal movement patterns in musculosketal disorders. Presented at the Workshop at Kaiser Permanente Hospital, Los Angeles, 13–14 August

Kendall FP, McCreary EK, Provance PG (1993) Muscles: testing and function, 4th edn. Williams & Wilkins, Baltimore

Kenneally M, Rubenach H, Elvey R (1988) The upper limb tension test: the SLR test of the arm. In: Grant R (ed) Physical therapy of the cervical and thoracic spine. Churchill Livingstone, New York, pp 167–194

Klein-Vogelbach S (1990a) Functional kinetics. Springer, Berlin Heidelberg New York

Klein-Vogelbach S (1990b) Ballgymnastik zur Funktionellen Bewegungslehre, 3rd edn. Springer, Berlin Heidelberg New York

Klein-Vogelbach S (1990c) Functional kinetics: Swiss ball videotape. Springer, Berlin Heidelberg New York

Klein-Vogelbach S (1995) Gangschulung zur funktionellen Bewegungslehre. Springer, Berlin Heidelberg New York

Lord S, Castell S (1994) Effect of exercise on balance, strength and reaction time in older people. Aust J Phys Ther 40:83–88

Lord SR, Clark RD, Webster IW (1991) Physiological factors associated with falls in an elderly population. JAGS 39:1194–1200

MacRae PG, Lacourse M, Moldavon R (1992) Physical performance measures that predict faller status in community-dwelling older adults. J Orthop Sports Phys Ther 16(3):123–128

Maitland GD (1986) Vertebral manipulation, 5th edn. Butterworths, London

Maitland GD (1992) Peripheral manipulation, 3rd edn. Butterworth-Heinemann, Oxford

Medical Research Council (1978) Aids to examination of the peripheral nervous system. Memorandum no 45. Pedragon, Palo Alto

Perry JP (1992) Gait analysis. Slack, Thorofare

Tinetti ME, Ginter SF (1988) Identifying mobility dysfunction in elderly patients. JAMA 259:1190–1193

Travell JG, Simons DG (1983) Myofascial pain and dysfunction: the trigger point manual. Williams & Wilkins, Baltimore

Travell JG, Simons DG (1992) Myofascial pain and dysfunction: the trigger point manual, vol 2. Williams & Wilkins, Baltimore

Umphred DA (1995) Classification of treatment techniques based on primary input systems. In: Neurological rehabilitation, 3rd edn. Mosby, St. Louis, pp 118–178

Weiner DK, Duncan PW, Chandler J, Studenski SA (1992) Functional reach: a marker of physical frailty. J Am Geriatr Soc 40:203–207

Whittle MW (1991) Gait analysis. Butterworth-Heinemann, Oxford

Wu G (1994) A review of body segmental displacement, velocity, and acceleration in human gait. In: Craik RL, Oatis CA (eds) Gait analysis. Mosby, St. Louis, pp 205–222

8 Assistive Devices

OBJECTIVES

By the end of this chapter the reader will be able to:
- Select assistive devices when exercising with the Swiss ball
- Increase trunk stability using assistive devices
- Challenge balance using assistive devices
- Increase strength using assistive devices
- Use the Swiss ball as an assistive device for manual therapy

New assistive devices are available that can be used in combination with the Swiss ball to enhance proprioceptive training and challenge balance. Other assistive devices, such as dumbbells and Thera-Band, have been available for many years. In combination with the Swiss ball they make exercises more challenging and help to increase stabilization. Assistive devices can enhance stabilization, proprioceptive training, challenge balance, and increase body awareness and strength. The following assistive devices are described below: (a) Sitfit, (b) foam roll, (c) Thera-Band, and (d) dumbbells.

8.1 Sitfit and Swiss Ball

Chapter 7 describes the use of the Sitfit in combination with the Swiss ball to challenge and test balance. There are many other ways to use the Sitfit, both with and without the Swiss ball. It is probably used the least to "sit fit"!

Lying on three Sitfits was not explored in Chap. 7. Have the patient lie in supine position on three Sitfits placed under the head, shoulder girdle/thorax and the lumbar spine/pelvis. The legs are supported by a Swiss ball while the arms are elevated so that there are no fixed points of contact with the environment.

> Substantial trunk stability is required to stay on this mobile surface.

The abdominal, back extensor, and hamstring muscles (as well as other muscles of the extremities) work reactively. The challenge is great. Because the patient cannot fall, he feels safe to practice.

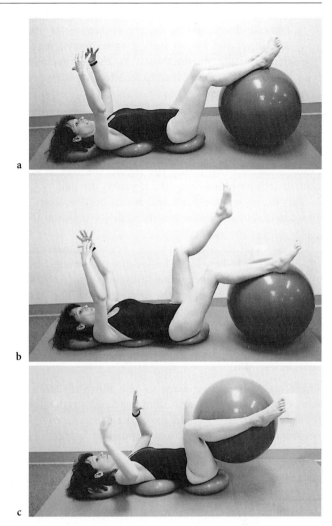

Fig. 8.1 a. Starting position for exercises on three Sitfits with legs on the Swiss ball. **b.** Lifting one leg off the Swiss ball with arms elevated while resting on three Sitfits. **c.** Lifting the Swiss ball with both legs while stabilizing the trunk on three Sitfits.

EXAMPLES

Figure 8.1. Panel a. The starting position. Before assuming this position, as a variation, the patient could rest both arms and one leg on the floor, then lift one leg or one arm, both arms and keep one leg on the floor, etc.

Panel b. Three extremities must be held by the trunk, which is lying on three Sitfits. This demands great concentration and quick reactions of the involved muscles.

> Because the weight of the three extremities must be stabilized against rotational and lateral flexion movements, it can be assumed that the deeper trunk muscles such as the semispinalis, multifidi-, rotatores and intertransversarii muscles are also activated in addition to the abdominal muscles.

As the patient performs this exercise, the therapist compares the two sides for strength and skill. For many patients the concentric activity of the hip flexor muscles when lifting the leg off the ball is more difficult than the eccentric activity of lowering the leg onto the ball.

This exercise can be fun and trains body awareness in both older children and adults, but it may be too difficult for children under the age of 5 years.

> **EXAMPLES**
>
> Figure 8.1. Panel c. The weight of the legs, arms and the Swiss ball hangs on the abdominal muscles, which are already actively keeping the trunk stable on the three Sitfits. The activity of the hamstring muscles at their distal attachment promotes a posterior tilt of the pelvis and helps to keep the lumbar spine flat, preventing an evasive movement of the spine into lumbar extension.

There are many more ways to use the Sitfit under the trunk, hands and knees, some of which are demonstrated in the following section with the foam roll. Therapists could make the exercises even harder by giving manual resistance with one finger, gently pushing against the arms, or one leg.

> The ball requires immediate automatic responses if the patient is to stay in the state of balance.

8.2 Foam Roll and Swiss Ball

> Foam rolls are used in physical therapy to train trunk stability, perform balance exercises, and mobilize the spine.

They consist of compressed foam of the sort used for insulation of pipes and for floating devices in swimming pools. The foam roll was first used with patients by Parker (1992), who is a physical therapist practicing the Feldenkrais approach; she has since produced two video tapes on the use of the foam roll (Parker 1993, 1995).

> *Caution:* Therapists should be aware that horizontal activities require a different programming of the central nervous system than do vertical activities. Therefore it is important to switch to a functional activity and practice there once the mobility and strength have been achieved in the contrived environment.

Selection of Foam Rolls. If possible, it is best to keep three different sizes of foam rolls available, with diameters of approximately 8, 10, and 12 cm and to cut sections the approximate length of a trunk (ca 1 m). Because the foam roll is easy to cut, the therapist can cut slices off a roll as necessary, for example, as support for the head. Another possibility is to cut the foam roll lengthwise. To add stability (and comfort) the patient can then rest on the flat surface with the back or place the feet on the wider surface.

EXAMPLES

Figure 8.20. A cut foam roll is placed alongside the Swiss ball to prevent it from rolling sideways. The small-diameter foam roll is very useful for self-mobilization of the spine (Adams 1995; Parker 1995; Carrière 1996). All sizes of the foam rolls are frequently used in combination with the Swiss ball.

Figure 8.2. Panel a. The patient's head and trunk are supported on a foam roll, both arms act as stabilizers, and one foot is on the Swiss ball. The weight of the other leg, which is held up in the air, needs to be stabilized by the trunk.

Panel b. The patient lifts the right leg and the left arm, a movement which decreases his BOS. This increases the instability of the position demanding more reactive trunk control.

Panel c. Only one foot is resting on the floor, while the ball is held by both arms. The weight of the right leg, the ball, and both arms must be stabilized by the trunk on the unstable foam roll.

Figure 8.3. Use of the medium-sized foam roll destabilizes the BOS under the hands, causing the shoulder girdle to stabilize while the abdominal and the hip flexor muscles pull the extended legs under the trunk. There are no stable points of contact with the environment. This exercise is adapted from the exercise "Sea Urchin" (Klein-Vogelbach 1990a,b; see Sect. 9.14).

Figure 8.4. This exercise demands concentration, skill, coordination, balance, and good strength of the muscles of the trunk and the extremities. There are no stable points of contact with the environment. The exercise is more difficult than the one in Fig. 8.3 because the Swiss ball is under the forearm, and the ball rolls more easily than the foam roll under the knees. The Swiss ball must be prevented from rolling away, and the bridge between elbows and knees is rather large. To make the exercise easier the patient should begin with a smaller bridge construction.

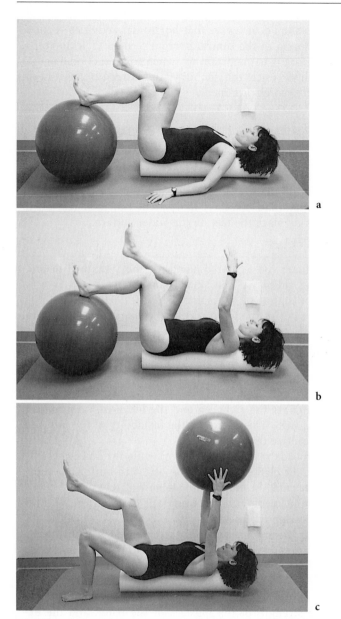

Fig. 8.2 a. Stabilizing the trunk on a large foam roll (approximately 10 cm diameter) with one leg in the air and both arms on the floor. **b.** Same as in **a.** but with right leg and left arm elevated. **c.** Both arms are holding a Swiss ball, one leg is elevated while the trunk is balancing on the foam roll.

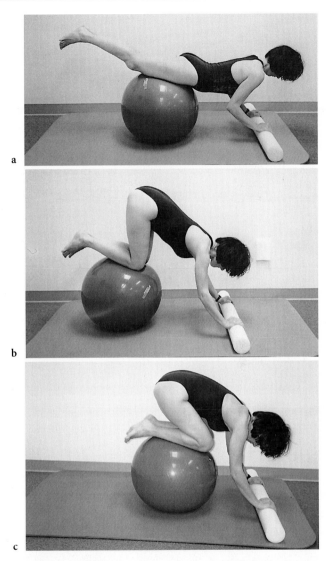

Fig. 8.3a–c. The extended knees are pulling the Swiss ball under the trunk while the hands are balancing on a foam roll.

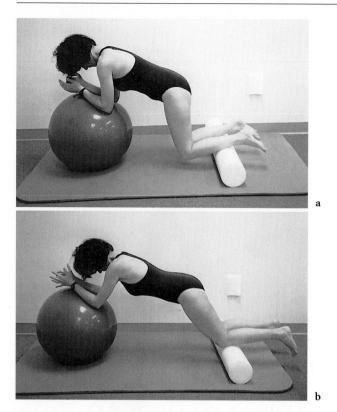

a

b

Fig. 8.4a,b. The Swiss ball must be pulled with the elbows toward the knees while the knees, resting on a foam roll, pull in direction of the elbows.

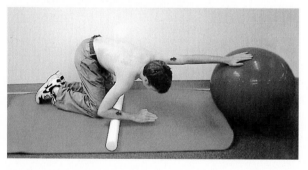

Fig. 8.5. A patient moves his arms into opposite directions using the foam roll and the Swiss ball.

Fig. 8.6. Great concentration is required while sitting on a Swiss ball, holding a foam roll between hands and knees and balancing with the feet on a Sitfit.

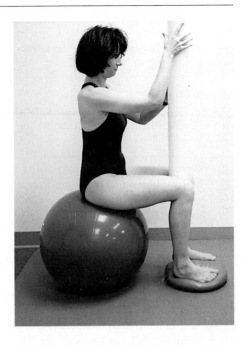

Figure 8.5. A patient with poor mobility of the spine uses the foam roll and the Swiss ball to facilitate movement of the arms in opposite directions, mobilizing the spine at the same time into extension and lateral flexion.

Figure 8.6. The Swiss ball, the Sitfit, and the foam roll are used together. Great concentration is required when sitting on a Swiss ball, holding a foam roll between hands and knees while balancing with the feet on a Sitfit. The trunk must maintain stability, and the extremities must stabilize at the same time that the points of contact with the environment are unstable. If the patient finds the exercise easy, the therapist can push on the shoulders, head, or the foam roll (using only the tip of the finger) or ask the patient to close his eyes (while being supervised).

8.3 Swiss Ball and Thera-Band

Thera-Band is an elastic band about 10 cm wide and color coded for its strength. It is used for many strengthening and stabilization exercises. Patients like to feel the resistance which the Thera-Band gives. Thera-Band can even be used by bed-bound patients since it can be attached easily to the frame of the hospital bed for the patient to practice. For such use, the therapist may want to cut Thera-Band into sections of approximately 1 m.

> In combination with the Swiss ball the Thera-Band adds stability and serves as a tool for resistive strengthening exercise (see also Chap. 14).

The following exercises serve as examples and should stimulate the reader to experiment with more exercises for the patient.

EXAMPLES

Figure 8.7. Panel a. The patient is in prone position over the Swiss ball pulling the Thera-Band apart with both elevated arms, strengthening the trapezius muscle while stabilizing the extended trunk on the Swiss ball. Notice the wide BOS of the feet. If the feet are placed closer together, the exercise becomes very difficult.

Panel b. The pull of the Thera-Band is diagonal: The left arm pulls into forward flexion, external rotation and abduction of the shoulder, and supination of the forearm. The right arm should be alongside the trunk in the midfrontal plane in extension, internal rotation and adduction with the forearm in pronation (and shoulder depressed).

The Brunkow concept supports exercises of this nature, except that Brunkow did not know of the Thera-Band (Bold and Grossman 1883). Very good to normal strength of the extensor muscles of the trunk and the muscles of the extremities is required for this exercise, as well as skill and coordination.

Panel c. The patient rolls the Swiss ball over the Thera-Band. The patient's body and left hand stabilize the Swiss ball while the right arm pulls into forward flexion and abduction using the Thera-Band.

Figure 8.8. A patient who had poliomyelitis in his right lower extremity is strengthening the leg with the "Valerie" exercise. This exercise was named after a young girl with a severe patella-femoral problem, aggravated by a very weak vastus medialis of the quadriceps muscle and poor alignment of one lower extremity.

She had great difficulty at first performing the exercise "invented" for her. "My muscles never worked so hard," she often exclaimed. Holding a sheet (for motivational reasons called an imaginary $100 bill) under the base of the big toe forced the fore-foot to be activated into pronation. The heels were elevated to decrease the BOS and to strengthen the calf muscles. The Thera-Band encouraged the patient to keep the knees apart. When a string was used instead, the patient was not allowed to drop the string.

The Valerie exercise has become a standard exercise for many patients who require correction of lower extremity alignment and strengthening of the vastus medialis muscles of the quadriceps and for patients with weak lower extremity muscles.

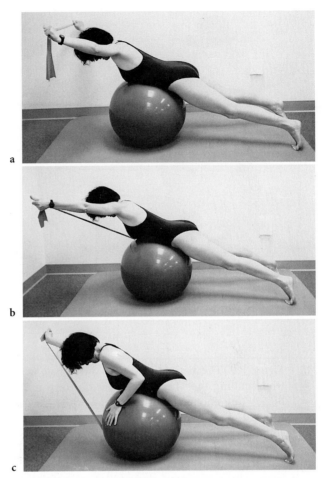

Fig. 8.7a. The Swiss ball and Thera-Band used in prone position challenging the back extensor and trapezius muscles. **b.** The patient is pulling diagonally. The left arm moves into forward flexion and abduction, the right arm into extension and adduction of the shoulder. **c.** The weight of the trunk on the ball holds the Thera-Band, and the right arm pulls into forward flexion and abduction of the shoulder. The left arm stabilizes the Swiss ball.

Regardless of whether the patient sits still on the ball or bounces, he must hold the forefoot firmly planted on the floor.

The following two exercises serve as examples of the Swiss ball used in combination with the Thera-Band and the Sitfit. These exercises are of course a progression from sitting on a Swiss ball with both feet planted on the floor.

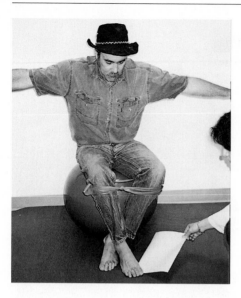

Fig. 8.8. A patient with decreased strength and proprioception of the right lower extremity keeps his forefoot pronated while sitting on the Swiss ball. The lower extremity muscles are activated in a closed kinetic chain while strengthening the hip abductors with Thera-Band.

EXAMPLES

Figure 8.9. The patient sits on a Swiss ball with both feet on a Sitfit while pulling the Thera-Band in a diagonal pattern. The left hand stabilizes one end of the Thera-Band while the right hand pulls it into forward flexion, slight abduction, and external rotation of the shoulder.

Figure 8.10. Each foot is placed on a Sitfit, while the patient sits on a Swiss ball and symmetrically pulls apart the Thera-Band above his head. These exercises obviously demand great activity from the legs as well as of the trunk and arms. All the muscle activities must be skillfully coordinated.

As a progression, the supervised patient can do the exercise with the eyes closed.

Other variations are also possible:

- Thera-Band can also be used attached to stall bars while sitting on a Swiss ball or lying prone over a Swiss ball. The two hands can pull either end of the attached Thera-Band downward from forward flexion of the arms into extension, etc.
- Wall pulleys can be used similarly to the Thera-Band in combination with the Swiss ball.
- Expanders have the same concept as the Thera-Band and can be used in a similar fashion with the Swiss ball.

Fig. 8.9. Combination exercise with the Sitfit, Thera-Band, and the Swiss ball to train strength, balance, and proprioception.

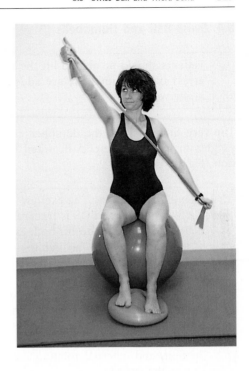

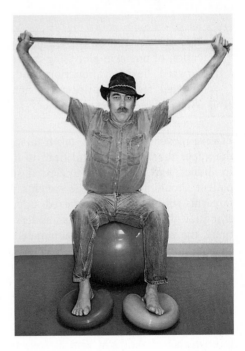

Fig. 8.10. Sitting on a ball, with two Sitfits under the feet, and with both arms elevated while pulling the Thera-Band. (The patient challenges proprioception, strength, and balance).

8.4 Swiss Ball and Dumbbells

> Patients should be able to lift the weight of the body segment (arm or arms) before dumbbells are added. It is most important not to use heavy weights.

The very fit model for the dumbbell exercises had great difficulty with 1-lb weights in her hands especially when lifting both dumbbells in prone position (Fig. 8.11a).

Figure 8.11. Panel a. The exercise is performed in prone position over the Swiss ball. The BOS is triangular with the feet wide apart. The patient should be able to lift both arms into the midfrontal plane before lifting weights. It is helpful to instruct the patient to stabilize the shoulder girdle by pulling the shoulder blades actively medial and caudally.

Panels b, c. Dumbbells are used while in lying supine position on a Swiss ball. The BOS is wide and the arms move in a diagonal pattern. The left arm is stabilized in extension and adduction and internal rotation of the shoulder, the right arm moves from forward flexion, abduction, and external rotation diagonally into adduction and pronation to the left hip

> The exercise can be carried out by holding a weight (1 lb) for stabilization of one arm alongside the trunk and moving the other arm into forward flexion, abduction, and external rotation. The pattern is adapted from proprioceptive neuromuscular facilitation (Knott and Voss 1968; Adler et al. 1993).

Evasive movements that are taken to shorten the lever to be lifted may cause the upper thoracic spine and head to flex, the shoulders to elevate, the arms to abduct, and the elbows to flex. If such evasive movements do occur, the patient should try to lift the weights with a short lever, for example, with forearms supinated, elbows flexed, upper arms adducted in midfrontal plane alongside the trunk, and the shoulders retracted. If evasive movements continue, the weights should be eliminated. Evasive movements do not train the correct muscles, and are easily recognizable because they lack harmony.

The therapist should remember that both arms are in an open kinetic chain in a free play function (see Chap. 6). The activity of the muscles is primarily on the superior surface of the arm and therefore continuously changes from the starting position in Fig. 8.11a to the end position in Fig. 8.11b. The trunk must stabilize the constantly changing lever (and therefore weight) of the right arm as well as the weight of the left arm. The hip extensor muscles are activated against gravity while bridging.

Fig. 8.11 a. Prone over the Swiss ball lifting 1-lb dumbbells against gravity. **b.** Supine on the Swiss ball (using dumbbells) diagonal arm pattern, the left arm is in extension, the right arm in forward flexion, abduction, and external rotation. **c.** Supine on the Swiss ball, dumbbells moved similar to the chopping pattern to the left side.

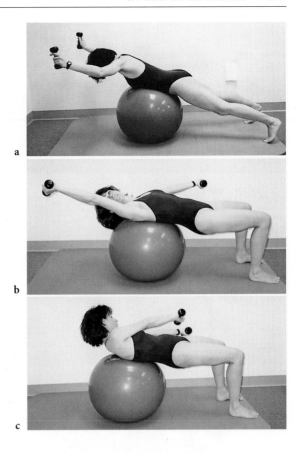

a

b

c

EXAMPLES

Figure 8.12. Two dumbbells are moved in a supine position in a diagonal pattern of proprioceptive neuromuscular facilitation. The goal of this exercise is to strengthen the abdominal and neck flexor muscles while keeping the pelvis and lower thoracic spine aligned. In the starting position both arms are elevated in forward flexion, slight abduction, and external rotation in the midfrontal plane above the head. The forearms in supination. The head is turned to look at the right hand.

The arms then move into approximately 90° flexion of the shoulders before reaching the end position with the arms adducted, internally rotated, and the forearms pronated. The head and upper thoracic spine move into flexion. This explains the slight evasive movement in panel c: The patient is extending rather than maintaining a neutral lumbar spine. The lower abdomen is lengthened rather than shortened. The head is flexed more than the upper thoracic spine. Overall, the movement lacks harmony. A patient should be instructed to do the exercise only in the range in which it can be done correctly.

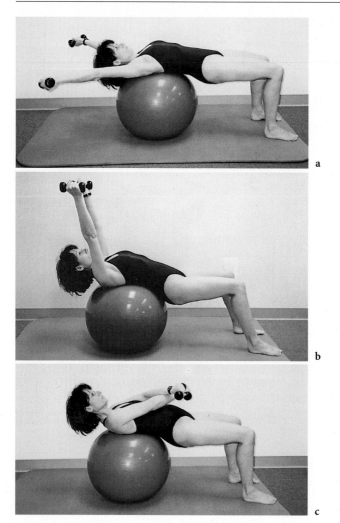

a

b

c

Fig. 8.12a–c. Bilateral arm pattern in supine on the Swiss ball with dumbbells. The direction of the arm movements is from forward flexion, abduction, and external rotation into extension, adduction, and internal rotation.

Obviously there are many more exercises that the patient could do using dumbbells while either sitting or lying in prone or supine position over the Swiss ball. The best way for the therapist to decide whether the patient can do the exercise safely is to try the exercises herself and analyze the muscle activity.

8.5 Swiss Ball as an Assistive Device in Manual Therapy

> Therapists trained in manual therapy regardless of which approach they apply know of the difficulties in finding the right position and exerting the ideal amount of traction or compression.

Numerous techniques have been recommended (Cyriax 1982; Greenman 1989; Kaltenborn 1989; Maitland 1986, 1992; Frisch 1995; Lewit 1992), but they all have a common goal: to mobilize tight structures of a joint with decreased motion. Some manual therapists use belts to fixate a body segment (Kaltenborn 1989). A difficulty often encountered by therapists is the discrepancy between the proportions of the patient and those of the therapist. For example, a small therapist may have a big patient who needs mobilization, distraction, or compression of a joint.

Uses of the Swiss ball include:
- The therapist can sit on it.
- The weight of the patient's body or a part of it can be supported by it.
- The patient can self-distract his spine with it.

> With the patient positioned in supine or prone position on a mat table or on the floor the therapist sits on a Swiss ball with a diameter of 55 or 65 cm (depending on the patient's leg length and on the mobility of the therapist). The therapist should sit at the level of the knees or more distal or proximal and place the patient's leg on her thighs.

Various starting positions are possible:
- The therapist can have one foot placed along the side of the trunk and the other foot placed at a right angle under the knees or lower legs of the patient.

> **EXAMPLES**
>
> *Figure 8.13.* The therapist demonstrates her mobility in at least four directions while the patient is pulling both legs into flexion and rotation. Because the weight of the patient's legs rests on the therapist's legs, the therapist has both her hands free to use for mobilization, compression, or distraction.
> (This position is also useful for PNF patterns of the lower extremities.)

- The therapist can sit on a larger ball with one knee and hip flexed to approximately 90° in front of the ball and her other leg extended at the hip with the foot placed behind the ball. This position is useful when the patient's foot is placed off the center of the ball, and the therapist wishes to mobilize the ankle which is restricted in dorsal flexion.

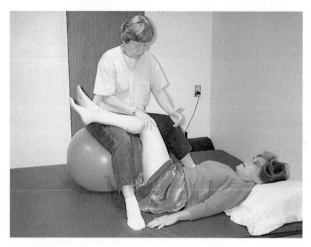

Fig. 8.13. Placing the patient's legs on the therapist's thighs frees the hands of the therapist for exercises and mobilization. This starting position makes the therapist mobile in at least four directions.

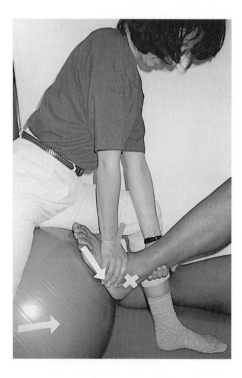

Fig. 8.14. Demonstration of dorsal glide of the patient's left talus to increase ankle movement of dorsiflexion.

EXAMPLES

Figure 8.14. The therapist applies pressure with her right hand in a dorsal direction mobilizing the patient's talus of his left foot.

- The therapist can sit on the ball at the level of the foot, knee, or hip, with both of her legs in front of the ball.

EXAMPLES

Figure 8.15. Panel a. The therapist has her hands free to perform traction combined with rotation at the knee.

Panel b. The therapist demonstrates compression and rotation of the knee bent at approximately 90° with the patient in prone position. This mobilization may be indicated with restriction of knee flexion, extension, or rotation.

Panel c. With the patient in supine position the therapist can mobilize the tibia or fibula in a dorsal direction. The patient's lower leg rests comfortably on the therapist's thighs. This mobilizing may also be indicated in patients with decreased flexion or extension of the knee or lack of dorsiflexion of the ankle. The therapist can also use this position for a ventral/dorsal glide of the femur in the hip joint.

Panel d. The therapist loops her arms around the patient's proximal lower legs. Each of the therapist's hands is placed on her other forearm. The elbows which are stabilized on her thighs are used as a fulcrum when performing distraction. Some anterior movement of the tibia at the knee may also take place although the femur is not stabilized at the knee joint.

In stabilizing the femur the positions in panels c and d can be used to test the laxity of the cruciate ligaments of the knee. The therapist could also have both of the patient's legs on her thighs and loop her arms around the patient's lower legs, again using her elbows to perform distraction, but this time of the lumbar spine. To achieve manual traction the therapist uses her feet to push onto the floor while holding on to the legs with her arms.

Figure 8.16. Panel a. The therapist sits on the ball with the patient's leg resting on her thigh. The position is used for compression or a dorsal glide of the femur in the hip joint at approximately 80° hip flexion.

Panel b. The therapist demonstrates distraction of the hip and knee joint with the patient in supine position. When the therapist pushes herself away from the patient with her feet, the ball rolls caudally. This distraction may benefit patients with decreased mobility of flexion and extension of the knee or hip joint and patients with unilateral lumbar spine or iliosacral joint problems.

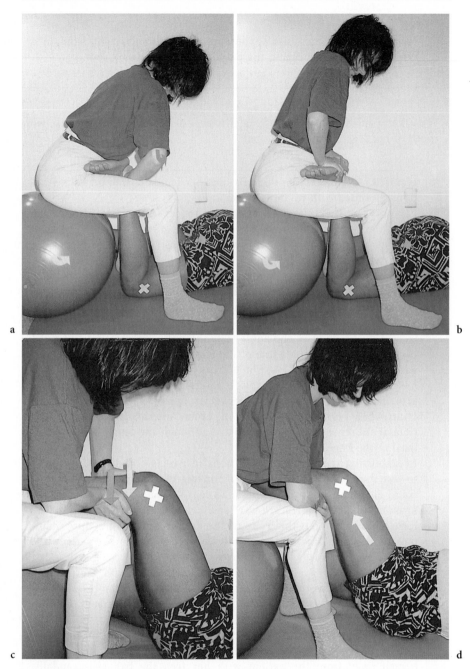

Fig. 8.15 a. The therapist has her hands free for traction and rotation at the knee joint.
b. The therapist performs compression and rotation at the knee joint. **c.** The therapist mobilizes the fibula into a dorsal direction. **d.** Looping the arms around the patient's lower leg,
the therapist uses her elbows as a fulcrum to achieve distraction at the hip joint.

Fig. 8.16 a. The therapist demonstrates compression/ dorsal glide of the femur in the hip joint. **b.** Distraction of the hip and knee joint can be performed with the patient in supine. **c.** The therapist's hands are placed on the patient's thigh to apply traction to the hip joint in prone position.

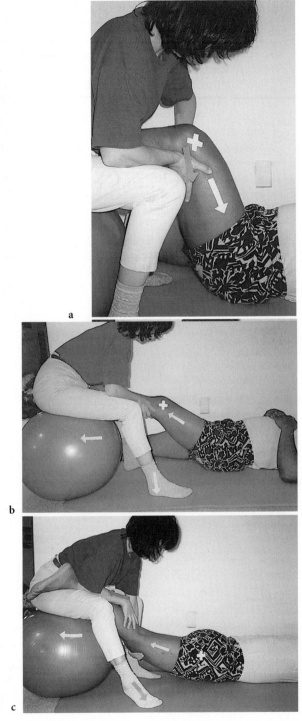

a

b

c

Panel c. The patient is in prone position, the therapist's hands are placed on the patient's thigh, and therefore only minimal traction takes place at the knee joint. Again, the therapist uses the ball as a medium to facilitate the distraction, which takes place at the hip joint. The patient's foot rests on the therapist's thigh. Mobility of the hip joint may increase with such distraction.

Figure 8.17. The therapist faces the side of the patient who sits cross-legged on the floor or at the edge of a mat table. The therapist demonstrates mobilization of the patient's right shoulder.

Panel a. The therapist applies pressure with her right hand to glide the patient's right humerus in a dorsal direction while fixating the scapula with her left hand. The patient's arm rests on the therapist's thigh and does not have to be lifted by the therapist.

Panel b. The therapist demonstrates a caudal glide of the patient's humerus combined with anterior rotation. Again, the therapist's left hand stabilizes the patient's scapula while her right hand moves his right humerus. Both mobilizations may improve movement of a stiff shoulder joint.

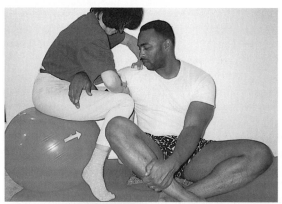

a

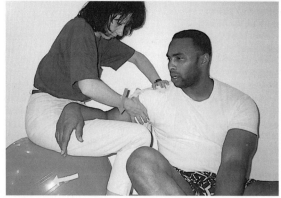

b

Fig. 8.17a. The therapist sits on the ball facing the side of the patient. While stabilizing the scapula with the left hand, the right hand performs a dorsal glide of the patient's humerus. **b.** The therapist demonstrates a caudal glide of the patient's right humerus combined with anterior rotation.

The therapist can use the same starting position or kneel behind the patient and place one hand on the scapula and the other on the anterior aspect of the patient's upper arm. When sitting at the side of the patient the therapist can push the ball away with her feet while stabilizing the scapula. The result is a buttressing (counter-) movement with distraction into abduction of the humerus at the humeroscapular joint. This movement prevents evasive movement of the scapula.

The same starting position is useful to free the hands to perform soft tissue mobilization of the anterior and posterior aspect of the shoulder and to move the humeroscapular joint in the frontal plane while ab- or adducting the humerus.

There are many possibilities of mobilizing the spine using the Swiss ball, sometimes in combination with the foam roll. Examples can be found throughout this book; a number are presented below.

EXAMPLES

Figure 8.18. The therapist stabilizes the patient's neck while the patient pulls his buttocks toward his heels, causing distraction of the cervical spine. The back is supported by the ball, which facilitates the distraction movement. It should be pointed out that some therapists have difficulty stabilizing themselves while sitting on a ball. In this case it may be better for the therapist to kneel or half-kneel behind the patient.

Figure 8.19. The therapist demonstrates mobilization into right lateral flexion and rotation of the thoracic spine and rib cage.

Figure 8.20. The therapist demonstrates mobilization of left lateral flexion of the thoracic spine combined with soft tissue mobilization of the rightside. This mobilization is easier on the double ball (PhysioRoll) because it cannot roll sideways. Here half a foam roll is placed next to the ball to prevent it from rolling to one side. The wall prevents rolling of the ball to the other side when a stretch is done without the help of another person.

Figure 8.21. A patient with decreased mobility of extension of the spine rests his feet on the Swiss ball. The patient can extend his back over the foam roll from this starting position. The roll can then be placed at different levels of the spine.

Extension of the spine can be mobilized many different ways: the ball can be placed against the wall behind a standing patient (Fig. 12.1h), the therapist can sit behind the patient as in the exercise "Sea Gull," (Fig. 9.6) or the patient can be in prone position over the Swiss ball as in the "Figurehead" (Fig. 9.18; Klein-Vogelbach 1990a,b).

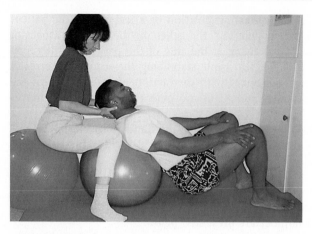

Fig. 8.18. The therapist stabilizes the patient's neck while the patient moves the ball to distract his spine.

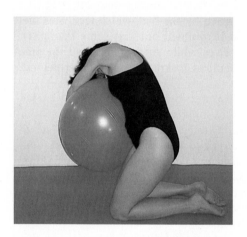

Fig. 8.19. The therapist demonstrates self-mobilization of the left of the spine/ribs into flexion/rotation to the right side.

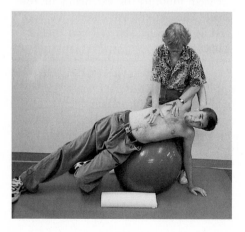

Fig. 8.20. Demonstration of left lateral flexion of the thoracic spine combined with soft tissue mobilization right side.

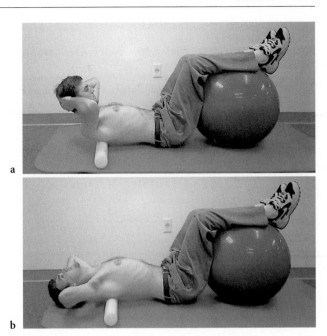

a

b

Fig. 8.21a,b. Self-mobilization of flexion and extension of the thoracic spine using the foam roll and the Swiss ball for positioning.

> The idea of using the Swiss ball for mobilization remains the same: It helps the patient to mobilize himself, and it helps the therapist to facilitate movements, frees the therapist's hands, and reduces the weight of the body segments which otherwise must be lifted. The examples given above provide the therapist with more possibilities of applying the Swiss ball while performing manual therapy.

References

Adams RC (1995) Patient compliance on a roll with foam. Adv Phys Ther 6:20–21

Adler SS, Beckers D, Buck M (1993) PNF in practice. Springer, Berlin Heidelberg New York

Bold RM, Grossmann A (1983) Stemmführung nach R. Brunkow. Enke, Stuttgart

Carrière B (1996) Therapeutic exerciser and self-correction programs. In: Flynn TW (ed) The thoracic spine and rib cage. Butterworth-Heinemann, Boston, pp 287–307

Cyriax J (1982) Textbook of orthopaedic medicine, 8th edn. Baillière Tindall & Cassell, London

Frisch H (1995) Programmierte Therapie am Bewegungsapparat. Springer, Berlin Heidelberg New York

Greenman PE (1989) Principles of manual medicine. William & Wilkins, Baltimore

Kaltenborn FM (1989) Manual mobilization of the extremity joints, 4th edn. Norlis, Oslo

Klein-Vogelbach S (1990a) Ballgymnastik zur Funktionellen Bewegungslehre, 3rd edn. Springer, Berlin Heidelberg New York

Klein-Vogelbach S (1990b) Functional kinetics: Swiss ball videotape. Springer, Berlin Heidelberg New York

Knott M, Voss DE (1968) Proprioceptive neuromuscular facilitation patterns and techniques. Harper & Row, New York

Lewit K (1992) Manuelle Medizin, 6th edn. Urban und Schwarzenberg, Munich

Maitland GD (1986) Vertebral manipulation, 5th edn. Butterworths, London

Maitland GD (1992) Peripheral manipulation, 3rd edn. Butterworth-Heinemann. Oxford

Parker I (1992) Beyond conventional exercises. Phys Ther Forum 7:4-7

Parker I (1993) Functional exercise program. I. Balance video. Ilana Parker Physical Therapy Service, San Francisco

Parker I (1995) Functional exercise program. II. Stretching and self mobilization Video. Ilana Parker Physical Therapy Service, San Francisco

9 Exercise Descriptions

Most of the exercises described in this chapter were developed by Klein-Vo-gelbach (1990a) on the basis of her functional kinetics concept (Klein-Vogel-bach 1990b). Klein-Vogelbach has presented a thorough analysis and a de-tailed description of each of the exercises (1990b) as well as a video tape of them, which is available in the United States (Klein-Vogelbach 1990c).

Although Klein-Vogelbach's exercises may initially appear too difficult for patients with medical conditions, the actual problem is generally that the therapist does not know the exercises and their purposes well enough to make the necessary adaptations for the individual patient's condition. All of Klein-Vogelbach's exercises should be considered *models of exercises which need adaptations*. The purpose in describing the exercises is thus to familiar-ize therapists with the original exercises of Klein-Vogelbach. The present de-scription and analysis highlights some important aspects of the exercises and provides some additional interpretations (Carrière 1993).

The following exercises have been developed by the author while working with patients in the hospital: "Stretch Myself" (Sect. 9.5), "Sea Gull" (9.6), "Walking On Hands" (9.16), "Push Me–Pull Me" (9.17), "Rock'n Roll" (9.24), and "Move My Legs" (9.25). The considerations when performing these exer-cises are the same as for all exercises with the Swiss ball and are described in Chaps. 4–7. To maximize the potential for carryover from exercises with the Swiss ball once the programs are established, a functional activity with-out a ball should follow.

> **OBJECTIVES**
>
> By the end of the chapter the reader will be able to select exercises for:
> - Stabilization of the spine
> - Mobilization of the spine
> - Postural training
> - Abdominal training
> - Hip mobilization and stabilization
> - Pregait training
> - Alignment of foot-knee hip
> - Reactive steps

Functional kinetic exercises with the Swiss ball have either a constant location, where the ball and the patient maintain the same or very similar base of support (BOS), or a changing location, where both the Swiss ball and the patient have an altered BOS at the end of the exercise.

EXAMPLES

Constant location: leaning backward and forward when sitting on a ball (see the "Scale," Sect. 9.2) or shifting the weight from the hands to the feet when leaning prone over a ball ("Swing," Sect. 9.10).

Changing location: the exercise "Sea Urchin" (Sect. 9.14) consists of the patient initially sitting on his heels on the floor but ending up on top of the ball, with the patient supporting himself with his hands on the floor.

The following descriptions of exercises explain the objectives, starting position, and actio. The latter is the initial (primary) movement which brings the patient toward the goal. It can be slow or fast (see also Chap. 6). The actio results in a reactio which is the spontaneous reaction of the patient to regain his balance and to prevent falling. Sometimes the patient must find a new BOS. Also presented are the conditios – instructions for the exercise to be carried out correctly, for example, recommendations for the speed of the exercises. Precautions and variations give special suggestions which may help the therapist to observe and instruct the patient with the exercises.

 Therapists should be aware of any contraindications and use their judgment to keep the patient safe from falls or injuries. Under no circumstances should these exercises cause any pain.

The following exercises begin with the patient sitting on the Swiss ball. The "Cowboy" is a good starting exercise and helps the patient become familiar with the Swiss ball.

9.1 "Cowboy"

Constant location exercise; Fig. 9.1.

Objectives
- To train for good upright posture that is automatic and economical
- To strengthen the quadriceps and calf muscles
- To prepare the patient for gait training
- To practice asymmetrical arm swing

Ball Size. The diameter of the ball should be slightly greater than the distance from the knee to the floor. Usually a 55-or 65-cm ball is required. The diam-

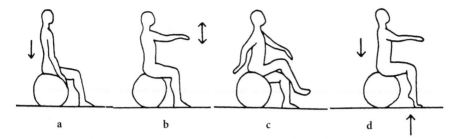

Fig. 9.1 a–d. The exercise "Cowboy".

eter needs to be greater if the patient has difficulties sitting 90°–90° at hips, knees, and feet.

Starting Position. Sit upright on the ball with both feet on the floor. The hips, knees, and feet are flexed at 90°. The knees and feet are hip-width apart. Weight bearing on the ball is centric (Fig. 9.1 a).

Actio. The primary movement for the patient is to push off the floor with the feet.

Reactio. The quadricep muscles are activated, and the trunk moves vertically, bouncing up and then down. The body must counteract the acceleration.

Conditio. The distance between symphysis pubis and sternal notch should not change during bouncing.

Speed. The ideal bouncing rate is approximately 120 bounces per minute for good dynamic stabilization of the spine at normal gait velocity.

Caution, Notes
- With an insecure patient use a slightly larger ball or begin on a Physio-Roll.
- When the ball is compressed by the body, expiration should not be blocked.
- Hyperactivity of the abdominal muscles can cause breathing problems.
- For safety the patient should keep the feet on the floor except for the variation with heel-lift.
- The patient should not lean forward or backward while bouncing.
- Vertical arm/hand movements can be added. If the push of the arms/hands is in a primarily downward direction, the back extensor muscles must reactively prevent trunk flexion. If the emphasis of the vertical arms/hands movement is in an upward direction, the abdominal muscles must prevent trunk extension (Fig. 9.1 b).
- The patient can shrug the shoulders to stimulate stabilization of the spine. The shoulder girdle must "drop" onto the stabilized trunk. This can also

- Patients with weak abdominal muscles tend to accelerate the movement where the muscles are weakest. The therapist should then emphasize training of the section of the movement where the acceleration takes place.
- The BOS can be decreased when the patient lifts the heels in the end position of the first actio. This makes the exercise more difficult.
- Insecure patients can do the exercise first on the PhysioRoll.
- During the exercise the arms can be moved in a sagittal plane, increasing the demand for stabilization of the trunk.

Examples
- A patient who has mastered maintaining trunk stability during the "Cowboy" and the "Scale" can progress to the "Indian Fakir" (Fig. 8.12, where dumbbells are uses in the end position).
- A patient who can align his feet and legs during the "Scale" exercise can progress to the "Indian Fakir." He now can see his legs at the beginning of the exercise only if a mirror is placed in front of him. When leaning back further he must take steps and keep the feet, lower legs, and thighs aligned without seeing them.

9.4 "Donkey Stretch Yourself"

Changing location exercise; Fig. 9.4. The main difference between this exercise and the "Indian Fakir" is that the hips flex when the patient leans backward. The patient progresses from sitting to leaning against the ball to lying on it.

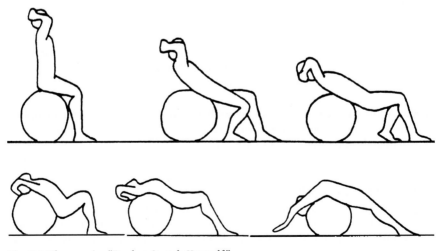

Fig. 9.4. The exercise "Donkey Stretch Yourself".

Objectives
- To mobilize the spine into extension, gravity assisted
- To stretch the ventral chain of the trunk
- To mobilize flexion of the spine against gravity
- To mobilize hip and knee flexion and extension
- To strengthen the lower extremities
- To train alignment of the lower extremities
- To practice reactive steps
- To stretch the pectoral muscles

Ball Size. Rather large to fit the extended back. Adaptations are necessary if the Swiss ball is too small, or the spine lacks mobility in extension (see Fig. 4.4).

Starting Position. Sit on the Swiss ball as in the "Cowboy", with the hands placed on the back of the head.

First Actio. The first movement is in the bridge: the ball rolls toward the feet, and the feet take steps forward to make room for the ball.

First Reactio. The point of body–ball contact changes from the ischium to the sacrum to the thoracic spine. The BOS increases.

Second Actio. The movement begins in the bridge, with the patient pushing the ball away with his feet.

Second Reactio. The knees, hips, and back extend when the patient lies in supine on the Swiss ball. Extending the arms above the head stretches the pectoral muscles and ventral chain of the trunk. The extension is gravity assisted.

Third Actio. The patient pulls the ball again toward the heels.

Third Reactio. The hamstring muscles are activated as well as the proximal gastrocnemius muscle when the feet pull the trunk to lean against the ball.

Fouth Actio. The patient returns to the starting position by pushing the ball away from the feet, taking steps backward and sitting up.

Fourth Reactio. The body–ball point of contact changes from cranial to caudal until the patient bears weight on both ischial tuberosities. There is concentric activity of the rectus femoris muscle, and the abdominal muscles are activated to achieve an upright position of the trunk.

Conditios
- The Swiss ball and feet should move in a straight line.

- At first the head should rest in the patient's hands or on a pillow to facilitate extension of the spine (Figs. 2.11b, 10.5d, 15.6a). (Extension of the spine is facilitated if the weight of the head does not have to be held by the neck flexor and abdominal muscles.)
- The legs should be in good alignment.
- For stretching of the pectorales muscles the arms should be elevated, slightly abducted in the shoulders, and the elbows extended.
- Weights can be attached to the patient's wrists for increased stretching of the pectoral muscles.

Speed. Comfortable speed, especially when changing back and forth from leaning to lying on the ball. There should be no unwanted acceleration during the different phases of the exercise.

Caution, Notes
- The head can rest on a pillow to decrease the strain on the ventral chain of muscles.
- A pillow can be placed under the low back to prevent hyperextension of the spine.
- The exercise lends itself to mobilization of the spine. The top of the ball acts as a fulcrum for the part of the spine which should be actively mobilized.
- Mobilization of active flexion against gravity can be combined with rotation of the thoracic spine.
- For greater stability this exercise can be done using a PhysioRoll.

Examples
- A patient who wants to mobilize the thoracic spine into flexion at approximately the 7th thoracic vertebra lifts his pelvis off the ball into a bridge activity to counteract (abut) the flexion movement initiated against gravity by the head, arms, and upper thoracic spine. The patient uses the ball as a fulcrum at approximately the 7th thoracic vertebra (or any other vertebra if it is positioned on top of the ball) while shortening the ventral chain. The patient can then move the head, arms, thoracic spine, and lumbar spine back into extension.
- A patient who has ankylosing spondylitis of his spine and hips wants to maximize the mobility of his hips and spine and strengthen his legs. The patient can work at the same time on aligning the legs as demonstrated in Fig. 11.13.
- A patient with multiple sclerosis obtains help from the therapist to learn balancing herself when moving from sitting to leaning on the ball (Fig. 7.22).

The following exercises are included because they have proven very useful in physical therapy practice. The first is named "Stretch Myself" because the patient is in control of the amount of stretching which takes place (see also

Fig. 8.18, demonstrating cervical distraction). The "Sea Gull" (so named because the arms resting on two balls resemble wings of a bird) is useful in mobilizing the back in extension while reducing the weight of the arms.

9.5 "Stretch Myself"

Constant location exercise; Fig. 9.5.

Objectives
- To achieve bilateral pectoral stretch
- To obtain single diagonal pectoral and trunk stretch
- To distract the spine with the patient in control of the amount of stretching
- To achieve soft tissue and neural tissue mobilization

Ball Size. Same size as with the "Cowboy," or larger if the patient has decreased mobility of the spine.

Starting Position. Supine over the ball as in "Donkey Stretch Yourself." The patient's arms are extended over the head, and the therapist stabilizes the arms by holding onto the patient's wrists, upper arms or even thorax or head.

Actio. The patient pulls his buttocks toward his heels.

Reactio. Self-stretch of the pectoral muscles, soft tissue mobilization anterior chest.

Conditios
- The therapist should not pull but rather only stabilize at the wrist, upper arms, trunk, or head.
- The patient must observe his pain limit to avoid overstretching.

Speed. Slow to allow for gentle pull; hold for 6–10 seconds in the end position.

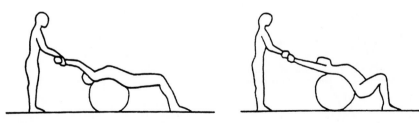

Fig. 9.5. The exercise "Stretch Myself".

Caution, Notes

- Avoid hyperextension of the cervical or lumbar spine in the starting position by placing pillows under the patient's head or hips.
- When pulling diagonally the patient pulls the left (right) buttock toward the right (left) heel.
- If the distraction of the spine is to be primarily in the lumbar region, the therapist should stabilize the patient's trunk with both hands.
- Some patients tolerate stabilization on the upper arm better than on the wrists.
- The symmetrical pectoral stretch and trunk distraction can be performed on a PhysioRoll.
- The patient can stretch neural structures of the upper extremities when holding onto a stall bar and pulling diagonally.

Examples

- A patient with poor postural alignment and a "tired" back after working all day feels relief by extending his back and distracting it with the help of a partner.
- A patient with decreased mobility of the pectorales muscle or tightness of neural structures in the upper extremity may want the diagonal stretch to gently mobilize all neural structures, similar to an upper limb tension test (ULTT) as described by Kenneally et al. (1988).

9.6 "Sea Gull"

Constant location exercise; Fig. 9.6.

Objectives

- To mobilize the spine into extension
- To facilitate weight shifting from side to side with elongation of the trunk
- To train balance and equilibrium reactions
- To reduce the weight of the arms

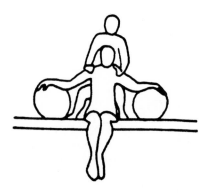

Fig. 9.6. The exercise "Sea Gull".

Ball Size. The therapist sits on a ball with a diameter approximately equal to the length of her lower leg. The ball under the patient's arm should be about 45–55 cm diameter, depending on the trunk and upper arm length of the patient.

Starting Position. The patient sits on the edge of a mat table, both posterior aspects of the thighs are in contact with the mat, and the lower legs hang over the edge. The patient's arms rest on top of two balls which are on either side of the patient. If the patient has decreased range of motion of one or both shoulders, the forearms are placed slightly off the center of the ball in less abduction of the shoulder. The therapist leans the patient's trunk forward to position the large ball close to the patient's back. The therapist sits on top of the ball behind the patient, her lower legs placed at the sides of the patient's trunk. The therapist's hands are placed at the anterior aspect of the axillae or on the shoulders.

Actio When Moving Forward. The therapist moves the ball with her buttocks closer to the patient's back while supporting the patient's shoulders/axillae and slightly pulling the shoulders and upper trunk upward and backward.

Reactio When Rolling Forward. Extension and distraction of the spine, anterior tilt of the pelvis.

Actio When Moving Sideways. The therapist moves the ball and the patient's trunk to the right (left) side.

Reactio When Moving Sideways. Elongation of the right (left) side of the trunk and increased weight bearing on the right (left) side of the buttock. Increased abduction of the right (left) shoulder.

Conditios
- The patient keeps his thighs in contact with the mat table throughout the exercise.
- The patient's back keeps contact with the ball throughout the exercise.

Speed. Slow and rhythmic.

Caution, Notes
- The exercise should not cause pain in the shoulders.
- If the therapist has long lower legs she needs to extend her legs more for the patient's comfort. The therapist's lower legs should be below the axillae of the patient (Figs. 11.27c, 13.21).
- The same exercise can be done with the feet resting on the floor. It provides a greater BOS but decreases equilibrium reactions of the lower extremities.

- The same starting position can be used for the patient to rotate the upper trunk and shoulder girdle while the therapist stabilizes the patient's head. This variation is helpful for patients who fear rotating their heads.
- In another variation the patient tries selective movements with the weak extremity which rests on a ball (Figs. 7.15d, 10.2f,g). Visual cues can be given by placing dots on the ball and having the patient observe and move the dots rather than actively extend or flex the arm.

Examples

- A patient with a whiplash injury to the neck who fears moving his head. Position him at the edge of a mat table and sit behind him on a Swiss ball. Place his arms on two smaller balls and gently support his head while he moves his arms on the ball in a circular direction and rotates the trunk. Later have the patient place his hands on his sternum and rotate the trunk while keeping the head still.
- With patients who have suffered a stroke the "Sea Gull" is very helpful in extending the spine, practicing weight shifting, and elongating the trunk while resting the arm on a ball. A reduction in muscle tone is often noticeable with a patient whose arms are on the Swiss ball.
- A patient with a "pusher syndrome." When the "pusher arm" is placed on a small Swiss ball, pushing is meaningless, and the therapist can work on posture and functional exercises to align the trunk and move the paralyzed arm.

9.7 "Hula-Hula, Forward/Backward"

Constant location exercise; Fig. 9.7. This exercise, which resembles the hula dance, trains small movements of the pelvis forward and back while the trunk remains spatially stable.

Objectives

- To mobilize the lumbar spine and hips in flexion and extension
- To promote automatic gait-typical movement of the lumbar spine and hips
- To train reactive stabilization of the thoracic spine
- To facilitate symmetrical arm swing

Ball Size. The same size as for the "Cowboy" exercise with firm pressure to promote easy rolling.

Starting Position. Sitting centrically on the ball, as in the "Cowboy" exercise. The arms can be placed on the chest or held in an oval above the head in the midfrontal plane.

First Actio. The ball is pushed away from the heels while the thorax remains stable in space (conditio).

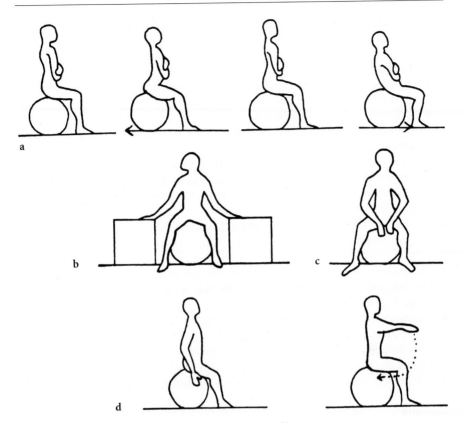

Fig. 9.7 a–d. The exercise "Hula-Hula, Forward/Backward".

First Reactio. Increase of lumbar lordosis, minimal displacement of knees into slight extension and feet into slight plantar flexion.

Second Actio. The patient should let the ball roll toward the heels without actively pulling the ball (to avoid hyperactivity of the abdominal muscles).

Second Reactio. Return to the starting position.

Conditios
- The distance between navel and xiphoid process should not change in order to stabilize the trunk (active buttressing, see Chap. 5).
- The distance between navel and symphysis pubis changes with each direction of rolling.
- The feet remain on the floor.
- If the symmetrical arm swing is added, the movement of each arm should be in a sagittal plane (Fig. 9.7 d).

Speed. Small movements backward/forward at approximately 120 times per minute (gait velocity).

Caution, Notes
- It is better to begin with extension of the lumbar spine to prevent hyperactivity of the abdominal muscles (Fig. 9.7 a).
- Breathing should not be blocked.
- The therapist can stand behind the patient and lift the trunk with both hands placed on the patient's rib cage.
- The patient can fixate the shoulder girdle by placing both hands right and left of the trunk onto two chairs. This lessens the weight of the trunk on the ball and the movement of the pelvis backward/forward is facilitated (Fig. 9.7 b).
- Placing the feet closer together diminishes the BOS and increases the equilibrium responses of hips and pelvis. This makes the exercise more difficult.
- The patient can place both hands on the ball between the thighs and resist the anterior/posterior movement of the ball while pushing it away with the heels (Fig. 9.7 c).
- Patients with hemiplegia can sit on a larger ball or PhysioRoll and place the upper extremities with the hands on the PhysioRoll next to the thighs to promote good weight bearing and ulnar/radial deviation of the hands during the backward/forward movement of the ball.
- For greater stability this exercise can be performed sitting on a PhysioRoll.

Examples
- Patients who have had surgery or a fracture of the lumbar spine, and who are allowed to move but are fearful. By supporting themselves with their arms on two chairs, the movement forward or back on the ball is easy to perform and usually very comfortable.
- Patients functioning at a higher level affected by a hemiplegia can learn to move their pelvis selectively.
- Patients with pelvic floor dysfunction can learn to move the lumbar spine and pelvis while breathing and keeping the thorax spatially fixed.

9.8 "Hula-Hula, Side to Side"

Constant location exercise; Fig. 9.8.

Objectives
- To facilitate lateral flexion of the lumbar spine at gait velocity
- To facilitate automatic equilibrium reactions
- To increase mobility of the pelvis/hips in the frontal plane
- To promote automatic gait-typical movements of the pelvis and hips in the frontal plane

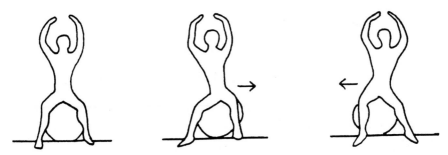

Fig. 9.8. The exercise "Hula-Hula, Side to Side".

Ball Size. The same as in the "Cowboy"; a larger ball is necessary if the patient's hip flexion is less than approximately 100°. The ball should be firm.

Starting Position. Sitting centrically on the ball as in the "Cowboy." The arms are elevated in an oval above the head in the midfrontal plane. If the feet are less than hip width apart, more equilibrium reactions are required and facilitated.

Actio. The ball begins to roll from side to side.

Reactio. The points of contact between ball and body change from both ischial tuberosities to one or the other.

Conditios
- The thorax remains "in place" (a spatially fixed point with only minimal displacement up and down).
- The distance between xiphoid process and navel does not change.
- The knees remain "in place" (spatially fixed points keeping the same distance between feet and knees).
- The ball should roll in a straight line from one side to the other side.

Speed. Approximately 120 repetitions per minute is preferable (gait velocity).

Caution, Notes
- A firm ball facilitates rolling.
- The therapist can hold and lift the patient's trunk slightly to decrease the weight of the trunk on the ball and facilitate the side to side movement.
- The patient can fixate his shoulder girdle by placing both hands right and left of the hips onto two chairs. The weight of the trunk on the ball is decreased, and the movement of the pelvis from side to side is facilitated (Fig. 11.22d).
- The patient can resist the side to side movement of the ball by placing the hands on the ball lateral of the patient's thighs.

Examples

- Patients recovering from surgery or fractures of the low back or hips who are allowed, but who are afraid to move may find this exercise helpful to begin moving, especially if the weight of the trunk is supported.
- Patients who have suffered a stroke, and who are ready to practice selective movements and weight shifting from side to side.
- Patients with pelvic floor dysfunction can practice movements and then progress to the exercise"Right Stop–Left Stop" (see Chap. 14).

The following five exercises have the same starting position, lying prone over the ball, but each has a different purpose. The exercises are contraindicated if the patient cannot lie on the stomach and cannot tolerate having the head down.

9.9 "Salamander"

Either constant or changing location exercise; Fig. 9.9.

Objectives

- To mobilize lateral flexion
- To stimulate weight shifting side to side
- To practice alternate weight bearing hands/feet of one side to the other side
- To switch between open and closed muscle activity of arm and leg of each side

Ball Size. The diameter of the ball should be approximately the length of the trunk. Slightly decreased pressure in the ball is more comfortable for the patient's stomach.

Starting Position. In prone position over the ball with the hands and feet "parked" (resting with their own weight only) on the floor. The arms and thighs "embrace" the ball. The trunk maintains contact with the ball throughout the exercise.

Actio. The arm and foot on one side push off to shift the weight to the arm and foot on the other side.

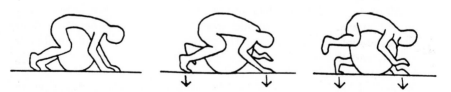

Fig. 9.9. The exercise "Salamander".

Reactio. When the push-off is initiated by the left arm and leg, the reactio is a closed kinetic chain (bridge activity) of the right arm and leg, while the left arm and left leg are in an open kinetic chain (free-play function). There is also a left side lateral flexion (side bend) of the trunk, with the spine concave on the left and convex on the right side of the trunk.

Conditios
- The trunk remains in contact with the ball at all times.
- The ball rolls in a straight line from one side to the other.
- Hands and feet should attempt to touch the floor at the same time.

Speed. A comfortable speed so that the patient can smoothly perform 10–15 repetitions.

Caution, Notes
- The exercise can be done such that the patient "lands" on the forearm and knee of the same side. This increases the lateral displacement of the ball and increases the lateral flexion.
- The speed can be increased to practice weight shifting.
- Patients with decreased mobility of the spine or long extremities need a bigger ball.
- The patient can increase the lateral flexion of the trunk and neck by looking toward the knee on the concave side.

Examples
- As a progression from the previous exercise.
- A patient who favors one side when weight bearing. He can practice shifting his weight from one side to the other. Dots can be placed on the floor on the spot the patient should try to touch with each weight shift.

9.10 "Swing"

Constant location exercise, but can also be performed with changing location; Fig. 9.10.

Objectives
- To practice physiological compression and distraction of the spine
- To practice alternate weight bearing for both hands, then both feet

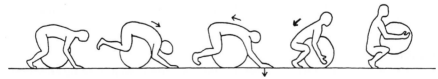

Fig. 9.10. The exercise "Swing".

Speed. Approximately 5 seconds per movement, or the rate of quiet breathing. The exercise can be coordinated with inspiration and expiration.

Caution, Notes
- The exercise should not cause any pain.
- The therapist can manipulate the ball or the pelvic movement.
- When mobilizing, the feet keep in contact with the floor throughout the exercise.
- When stabilizing, the weight of the legs and the pelvis must be held by the low back as soon as the feet lose contact with the floor.
- The therapist can give manual resistance with one hand placed on the sacrum and the other on the low back of the patient.
- The therapist can use the previous position for soft tissue mobilization by placing her hands crosswise on the sacrum and the lumbar spine and exerting mild pressure/stretch combined with rotation of the heel of the hands.
- The exercise can be used to train the pelvic floor muscles.

Examples
- All patients who need to learn tilt their pelvis anterior/posterior.
- Patients who have difficulty stabilizing the low back when lifting. Progress to giving resistance at the sacrum after the patient can tilt the pelvis anteriorly with the feet off the floor.
- A 9-year-old girl with an atonic bladder after a cauda equina syndrome combines the "Duck" exercise with breathing and back extensor training (lifting the arms against gravity) while activating the pelvic floor. The actio/reactio is combined with inspiration and relaxation, the return actio/reactio with exhalation and tightening of the the pelvic floor muscles (p. 259).
  The following exercises also begin in prone position.

9.12 "Crab"

Constant location exercise; Fig. 9.12.

Objectives
- To activate rotator muscles of the spine

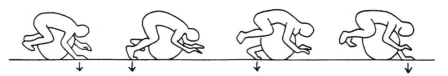

Fig. 9.12. The exercise "Crab".

- To practice coordination of the hands and feet
- To practice alternate weight bearing of the extremities

Ball Size. The same as in the "Salamander," but less pressure (for comfort).

Starting Position. Same as in the "Salamander."

Actio. Push-off from one point of contact with the floor to the next point of contact with the floor in the following order: left hand to the right hand, right hand to the right foot, right foot to the left foot, left foot to the left hand. Then change to the other direction.

Reactio. Clockwise or counterclockwise weight bearing of only one extremity at the time (three extremities must be stabilized/held by the spine).

Conditio. The trunk and upper arms remain in contact with the ball throughout the exercise.

Speed. Rather fast. If performed too slowly and the patient "thinks" too much, he usually fails.

Caution, Notes
- The exercise is usually well tolerated by patients with back pain because the trunk is supported.
- The patient must be able to tolerate the head-down position.

Examples
- Neurological patients functioning at a high level (such as after a head trauma or stroke) find both the "Crab" and the "Trot" challenging for weight bearing and coordination.
- Older children who need to work on balance and coordination.

9.13 "Trot"

Constant location exercise; Fig. 9.13.

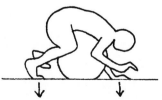
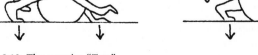
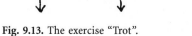

Fig. 9.13. The exercise "Trot".

Objectives
- To train diagonal weight bearing on one hand and the opposite foot
- To stabilize spinal rotation
- To improve coordination of hands and feet

Ball Size. The same as in the "Salamander."

Starting Position. The same as in the "Salamander."

Actio. Vertical push-off from the left hand and the right foot and then from the right hand and the left foot.

Reactio. With each weight bearing change, the weight of the other leg and arm must be stabilized by the trunk.

Conditios
- Trunk, upper arms and thighs remain in contact with the ball throughout the exercise.
- The patient should land each time with hand and foot on the same spot on the floor.
- There should only be vertical movement of the ball, no forward/backward movement.

Speed. Approximately 120 times per minute (gait velocity).

Caution, Notes
- Stop if the exercise is not well tolerated by patient (complaints of nausea).
- The exercise can be practiced first on all fours without the ball to achieve good coordination of hands and feet.
- When the knees are placed close together, there is less weight shifting from one side to the other.
- When the knees are placed apart, more weight of one leg and part of the pelvis must be stabilized because of the longer lever. This may also result in more unwanted weight shifting from side to side.

Examples. See previous exercise.

9.14 "Sea Urchin"

Changing location exercise; Fig. 9.14.

Objectives
- To mobilize the spine in flexion
- To achieve total flexion of knees, hips and the spine
- To practice weight bearing of both upper extremities

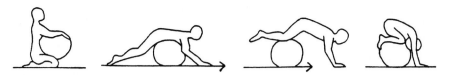

Fig. 9.14. The exercise "Sea Urchin".

- To practice forward flexion of the upper extremity in a closed kinetic chain
- To strengthen the abdominal muscles
- To train coordination and skill of the abdominal muscles

Ball Size. The diameter of the ball should be approximately the length of the patient's trunk.

Starting Position. Sitting on the heels, holding the ball on the thighs.

Actio. The trunk maintains contact with the ball while the patient first leans slightly backward, then thrusts himself forward prone over the ball and stops the forward movement with the hands when they reach the floor.

Reactio. When the hands reach the floor, and the weight of the shoulder girdle is supported, the knees and hips flex and pull the trunk under as soon as the thighs are on top of the ball (Fig. 11.12).

Conditios
- The ball rolls forward in a straight line.
- In the end position the patient is kneeling centrically on the ball with the hands flat on the floor (Fig. 11.12).

Speed. The ideal speed is reached when the patient, after accelerating the movement, does not overshoot the goal. The exercise should be practiced in slow motion first before accelerating.

Caution, Notes
- A patient with hip and/or knee flexion contractures cannot perform this exercise correctly.
- The exercise can be dangerous if the patient pulls the legs into flexion too early because he can roll off the ball.
- If the legs are pulled up too late, the patient ends off center on the ball.
- All points of contact change with this exercise.
- A patient with poor balance of the trunk muscles increases his BOS by keeping the knees and feet apart during the exercise.
- The exercise is more difficult when the feet and knees are placed close together.
- In the end position both hands remain flat on the floor.

- The exercise can be practiced leaning prone over a PhysioRoll, which adds stability.
- The exercise can be done in combination with a foam roll (see Fig. 8.3).
- Adaptations may be necessary for patients who have difficulty fully extending the wrists, such as those with carpal tunnel syndrome. In other patients it may help to stretch the neural structures, but the therapist must use her judgment of how much and how long to stretch the flexor muscles of the wrist.
- In the final position the knees can move the ball from side to side, adding rotation of the spine under the stable shoulder girdle. This variation is called the "Drunken Sea Urchin" (Fig. 12.1i). Skill and coordination (timing) of the abdominal muscles is required. This variation also causes horizontal ab- and adduction in the shoulder joints in a closed kinetic chain. The trunk moves on the stable shoulder girdle (spatial fixed point).

Examples. This exercise and the "Goldfish" are popular with both children and adults because they affect so many physical problems. Each is challenging for patients with shoulder and back problems or knee and hip flexion/extension deficits and for patients who need abdominal back extensor and hip flexor and extensor muscles strengthening, coordination and skill, as well as neural tension exercises. (See also Figs. 8.3, 11.21d, where it is used in combination with the foam roll.)

9.15 "Goldfish"

Changing location exercise; Fig. 9.15.
This exercise is usually performed in combination with the "Sea Urchin". After moving the body into total flexion, the "Goldfish" moves the spine, shoulders, hips, and knees into full extension (Fig. 11.20 a, b).

Objectives
- To practice total extension of the spine, hips, and knees
- To facilitate total forward flexion of the shoulders in a closed kinetic chain
- To strengthen back and hip extensor muscles

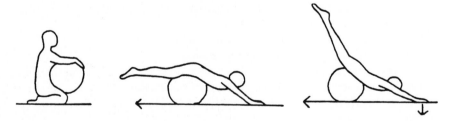

Fig. 9.15. The exercise "Goldfish".

Ball Size. The same as the "Sea Urchin."

Starting Position. The same as the "Sea Urchin" exercise. When the hands reach the floor, the following actio is initiated.

Actio. The hands remain planted on the floor; the arms extend and push the ball backward.

Reactio. The arms extend, the trunk moves backward, the hips and knees straighten, and the legs lift up in the air. The weight of the legs must be stabilized by the back and hip extensor muscles.

Conditios
- The hands keep in contact with the floor when the legs lift up.
- The ball rolls in a straight line.
- The low back should not hyperextend (observe the distance between xiphoid process and symphysis pubis to give proper instructions depending on the length of the trunk and extremities).

Speed. Slow enough so that the exercise can be done well and be held in the end position.

Caution, Notes
- The exercise requires good mobility of the hips and knees in extension.
- The patient should not overextend the lumbar spine.
- The exercise cannot be done correctly if the hands slide on the floor.
- The exercise can be adapted to mobilize shoulder flexion, the feet can then stay on the floor.
- The exercise can be done leaning prone over a PhysioRoll, adding stability.
- Resistance can be given at the feet of the patient for increased stabilization.
- The end position of the "Sea Urchin" can be the starting position of the "Goldfish."
- The "Mermaid" (Fig. 9.20) can be developed from this exercise.

Examples. The exercise is done on a Swiss ball and a PhysioRoll to evaluate and strengthen the hip extensor muscles (see Fig. 7.9).

The following exercise begins as the "Sea Urchin" or "Goldfish." It is useful to test the patient's trunk balance and upper extremity strength.

9.16 "Walking on Hands"

Changing location exercise; Fig. 9.16.

Objectives
- To prepare the patient for the exercises the "Sea Urchin" and the "Goldfish."

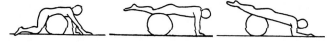

Fig. 9.16. The exercise "Walking On Hands".

- To stabilize the trunk
- To evaluate trunk balance
- To strengthen the upper extremities, especially the triceps brachii in a closed kinetic chain

Ball Size. Same as the "Sea Urchin."

Starting Position. Prone over the ball with the arms and feet parked as in the "Swing" exercise.

Actio. The patient walks forward on his hands.

Reactio. The feet leave the floor, the legs balance on the ball. The abdominal muscles work in a bridge activity.

Conditios
- The hands point forward; the elbows are not locked and point back toward the ball.
- Head and trunk remain in good alignment. The distance from the symphysis pubis to the xiphoid process should not change.
- The ball moves in a straight line.

Speed. Rather slow, to allow the patient to concentrate on the legs staying on the ball.

Caution, Notes
- The patient's hands should not be allowed to slide.
- The exercise is easier if the hands are kept in front of the shoulders.
- The demand on the triceps brachii increases if the shoulders are in front of the hands (Fig. 11.16b).
- The patient can perform push-ups, which are harder when the anterior bridge is larger (Fig. 11.16b).
- Alternate weight bearing can be practiced with the hands walking in place (Fig. 11.17b).
- The patient can rest the forearms on the floor and move the ball forward and backward to increase shoulder flexion and elbow flexion/extension (Fig. 12.1j).
- Patients with imbalances of the trunk (such as scoliosis) have difficulty keeping the feet on the ball.

- The exercise puts high demand on the abdominal muscles in a bridge activity when only be the feet remain on the ball.
- The exercise is much easier and requires less skill and balance when it is performed on the PhysioRoll. The BOS is increased, and the direction of rolling can only be forward and back (Fig. 11.17b).

Examples
- Patients with scoliosis find the exercise challenging.
- Patients who need to strengthen the upper extremities, especially the triceps brachii.
- Patients who need abdominal muscle strengthening.

9.17 "Push Me–Pull Me"

Constant location exercise; Fig. 9.17.

Objectives
- To strengthen the shoulder girdle/arm muscles concentrically and eccentrically

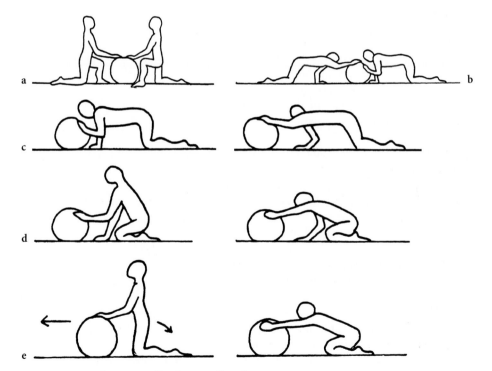

Fig. 9.17 a–e. The exercise "Push Me–Pull Me".

- To increase the range of motion in the shoulder joint
- To reduce the weight of the arm while exercising

Ball Size. As in the "Sea Urchin."

Starting Position 1 (Variation 1). Patient and therapist (or another patient) face each other half kneeling (trunk vertical) with their hands resting on the ball between them. The ball may be placed in various positions relative to the patient's body. (Fig. 9.17a; for other variations, see Figs. 13.2, 13.3.)

Actio. The therapist (or another patient) moves the ball forward/backward and side to side (concentrically) with the instruction to the patient to slow the movement without changing the hand position.

Reactio. The patient slows the movement eccentrically.

Conditios
- The patient's trunk should remain stable
- The hand does not move on the ball, only with the ball

Speed. Controlled and slow. When the therapist moves the ball suddenly and rapidly, the patient's ability to react quickly is trained.

Caution, Notes
- The exercise can be done while kneeling with one arm in approximately 90° forward flexion on the floor supporting the trunk (which is in a horizontal position in space; Fig. 9.17b, c)
- To increase the range of the shoulder flexion the movement can be practiced by the patient alone

Starting Position 2 (Variation 2). The patient begins in kneeling position (on both knees, trunk erect; Figs. 9.17d, e).

Actio. The patient moves the ball forward and at the same time the buttocks backward until sitting on the heels (Figs. 12.1b,c). This can also be done with two persons facing each other.

Reactio. Shoulder flexion from the proximal and distal lever with movement of the pivot point (humeroscapular) joint downward (Figs 9.17e).

Conditios
- Arms and pelvis/trunk move in opposite directions.
- The movement should not be forced.

Speed. Controlled, rather slow to allow for stretching.

Caution, Notes
- Resistance can be given or the ball movement can be slowed by another person.
- To increase the stretch the patient can add rotation by sitting at the side of the heels (Fig. 12.1d).
- The patient can begin by sitting on the heels and placing one hand on the floor and the other on the ball, while pushing the ball forward or forward and to the side of the supporting hand (variation 3).

Examples
- The exercise, developed in work with patients with shoulder injuries, is helpful for those with frozen shoulders and allows two patients to work together.
- A patient after a mastectomy with decreased range of motion of the shoulder (Figs. 12.1a–d).

9.18 "Figurehead"

Constant location exercise; Fig. 9.18.

Objectives
- To actively mobilize extension of the spine against gravity
- To stabilize the extended spine
- To strengthen the middle and upper trapezius muscles
- To strengthen the upper extremities in a open kinetic chain
- To strengthen the quadriceps muscle in a bridge activity

Ball Size. The same size as the "Sea Urchin;" larger if the patient has decreased mobility of the spine or long extremities.

Starting Position. Kneeling behind the ball, the trunk prone on the ball, and the hands in line with the shoulders on the ball.

Actio. The primary movement is from the hands, which push downward against the ball making it roll forward until the arms are extended. The pelvis is in contact with the ball (Fig. 9.18a).

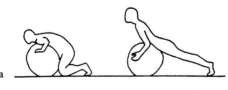

a   b

Fig. 9.18 a, b. The exercise "Figurehead".

Reactio. Extension of the spine against gravity. The knees extend in a bridge activity.

Conditios
- The feet remain planted with the extended toes on the floor.
- The ball rolls in a straight line.
- The lumbar spine should not overextend.

Speed. Depends on the amount of mobilization. If only small movements in several spinal segments take place the speed is approximately at gait velocity. The movement is slower if the patient extends the entire spine.

Caution, Notes
- The actio can be performed with the feet resting against a wall and pushing off from the wall (Fig. 11.11).
- The arms can hang down at first, and the patient rests on the ball with the sternum. When pushing off with the feet, the trunk extends, and the arms can be lifted into abduction and extension of the shoulders or into forward flexion (Fig. 9.18b).
- Insecure patients can practice the exercise first on the PhysioRoll.
- Insecure patients who practice on a ball tend to keep the feet apart or not extend their knees to increase the BOS.
- For increased stability the therapist can give gentle resistance to the arms in abduction or forward flexion, or to the head.
- The exercise is much harder with the feet and knees placed close together or one foot in front of the other.

Examples
- Patients with general weakness after a motor vehicle accident and poor alignment of the trunk and weakness of the upper and middle trapezius muscle improve their strength performing a modified version of the exercise (Fig. 7.14).
- The exercise is also used in patients with poor posture resulting from shortness of the pectoral muscles and weakness of the trunk extensor and upper and middle trapezius muscles (Fig. 11.21c).

9.19 "Scissors"

Constant location exercise; Fig. 9.19.

Objectives
- To facilitate trunk rotation under a stable shoulder girdle
- To strengthen the shoulder girdle in a closed kinetic chain
- To strengthen the hip abductor and adductor muscles in an open kinetic chain
- To stabilize the trunk extensor and rotator muscles

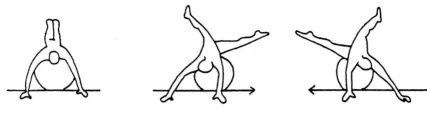

Fig. 9.19. The exercise "Scissors".

Ball Size. The same size as in the "Sea Urchin."

Starting Position. Lying prone over the ball with the hands placed approximately twice the width of the shoulder girdle from each other.

Actio. The primary movement begins with the gaze moving from one hand to the other as reading a scroll on an imaginary line between the hands.

Reactio. If the patient moves the gaze from the right hand to the left, the left half of the pelvis loses contact with the ball and must rotate counterclockwise so that he does not fall off the ball. The extended legs open in a step position with the upper (left) leg pointing upward and backward, the foot plantar-flexed, the lower (right) leg pointing downward and forward with the foot dorsiflexed.

Conditios
- The eye always keep the same distance from the floor.
- The hands remain firmly planted on the floor.
- The ball rolls in a straight line from side to side.

Speed. Comfortable speed so the patient can control the movement and no unwanted acceleration takes place. Later the patient can increase the speed of the exercise, which requires more equilibrium reaction, good strength, coordination, and timing.

Caution, Notes
- The exercise cannot be performed correctly if the hands slide.
- Patients with a heavy pelvis have more difficulty turning the pelvis from a horizontal to a vertical position in space.
- Patients with very good rotation of the trunk turn the pelvis later than patients with poor rotation of the trunk.
- The exercise must look harmonious; hyperextension of the lumbar spine should be corrected.
- For increased stabilization and strength, resistance can be given at the lateral side of the legs or at the heel of the upper leg and the dorsum of the foot of the lower leg.
- The "Mermaid" can be developed from the end position of this exercise.

Examples
- Patients 6 weeks after anterior cruciate reconstruction (see Chap. 11) can train skill and coordination of the hip extensor and ab- and adductor muscles (Fig. 11.10).
- Young patients recovering from a healed fracture of the spine who need to work on improving the rotation of the thoracic spine.

9.20 "Mermaid"

Changing location exercise; Fig. 9.20.

Objectives
- To practice lateral flexion of the trunk against gravity
- To strengthen the hip abductor muscles of the upper leg against gravity
- To stabilize the shoulder girdle in a closed kinetic chain
- To facilitate external rotation of the lower leg against gravity

Ball Size. The diameter is approximately the length of the thigh and the pelvis (when kneeling the top of the ball is as high as the iliac crest).

Starting Position. Half kneeling on the left knee with the right leg beside the ball at 90° hip, knee, and ankle flexion. The right hand rests on top of the ball, and the left hand rests on the right thigh. The body is positioned perpendicular to the direction of the ball's movement.

Actio. The primary movement begins with the right hand pushing the ball in a straight line to the right. The trunk and head lean to the right in a controlled fall until the right side of the trunk is in contact with the ball. Now the right foot pushes off and lifts upward.

Reactio. The ball continues to roll to the right until the hands stop the movement and make an anterior bridge. The (left) upper leg lifts (as a tentacle) into abduction of the hip; the (right) lower leg remains flexed and externally rotates in order to stabilize the left leg with the foot on the knee.

Return Actio. The ball is pulled toward the arms, and then the arms/hands push off.

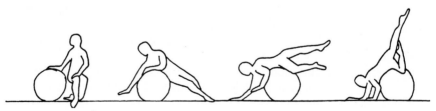

Fig. 9.20. The exercise "Mermaid".

Return Reactio. The ball moves in the opposite direction until the patient again reaches the starting position.

Conditios
- The frontal plane of the pelvis remains vertical in space throughout the exercise.
- The ball rolls in a straight line.
- Hyperabduction of the upper leg should be avoided.
- The thoracic and lumbar spine stay aligned in neutral flexion/extension.
- The right arm lands on the forearm, and the left arm rests on its left hand.

Speed. Slower when learning the exercise, since timing is critical.

Caution, Notes
- If the patient gets onto the ball too early, the ball touches the pelvis at the start of the exercise, and he tends to roll off (which can be dangerous!).
- If the patient gets onto the ball too late (the patient is hesitant and the ball too far away), the pelvis does not end on top of the ball.
- Long, heavy legs make balancing more difficult when the legs become a tentacle (Fig. 2.11c).
- A heavy pelvis and wide hips make it more difficult to keep the pelvis vertical in space.
- The exercise is contraindicated if hip contractures prevent neutral hip extension and more than 90° hip flexion.
- The exercise can be developed from the "Goldfish" and the "Scissors."
- The exercise is difficult, requires good timing and coordination, and should not be done by a novice.

Examples
- A young patient (after a healed fracture of the acetabulum) with weak hip abductor muscles who wants a more challenging exercise. The therapist would stand behind the patient and guide the movement with her hands at the patient's pelvis, until it is safe for the patient to do the exercise alone.
- Patients who need strengthening of the lateral trunk flexor muscles against gravity.

9.21 "Carrousel"

Changing location exercise; Fig. 9.21.

Objectives
- To practice weight shifting as typical in gait
- To train reactive steps
- To practice rotation around the longitudinal axis of the body
- To train skill and coordination

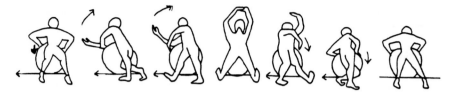

Fig. 9.21. The exercise "Carrousel".

Ball Size. The diameter of the ball should be the same as in the "Cowboy," at least half the length of the legs. A slightly larger ball facilitates the exercise as it increases the BOS and makes it easier for one leg to pass under the other leg, especially if the legs are long and heavy.

Starting Position. Lying prone on the ball with the hands on the ball below the shoulders. The trunk and the head are the tentacle, and the legs are extended and form a bridge. The feet are planted on the floor hip width apart. The toes are extended.

First Actio (Prone to the Right Side). The left hand pushes downward and makes the ball move to the left side.

First Reactio (Prone to the Right Side). The ball moves to the left side, the left shoulder moves back and upward, and the pelvis rotates at the same time counterclockwise. The right hand loses contact with the ball and moves forward and up.

Second Actio (Side to Supine). The left arm loses contact with the ball and moves backward in a transverse plane.

Second Reactio (Side to Supine). The right leg takes a step forward braiding under the left leg. The body becomes supine on the ball.

Third Actio (Supine to the Left Side). The arms continue to move in a transverse plane. Before lying on the left side the left arm lifts into forward flexion.

Third Reaction (Supine to the Left Side). The right arm crosses over midline, lands at shoulder level on the ball, and brakes the rolling movement of the ball.

Fourth Actio (From the Left Side to Prone). The left leg takes a step backward, braiding under the right leg.

Fourth reactio (From the Left Side to Prone). The right hand decelerates the side movement of the ball while the left hand is placed on the ball under the left shoulder. The trunk and pelvis rotate counterclockwise until reaching the prone position.

Conditios
- The ball should roll in a straight line.
- There should be no acceleration of the movement.

Speed. The speed must be slow enough for the movement to be controlled at all times (without any unwanted acceleration).

Caution, Notes
- Large hips or a small thorax make turning the body on the ball more difficult.
- Moving the ball more cranially facilitates turning for patients with large hips.
- If the step size is incorrect, the ball moves in a circle rather than a straight line.
- Each section of the exercise can be practiced separately.
- The exercise can be done in both directions.

Examples
- Patients with postural problems find this exercise challenging.
- A patient functioning at a high level after a head trauma who needs more training to coordinate the upper and lower extremities while turning the trunk in space.

The following Klein-Vogelbach exercises are carried out with the patient in supine position and are valuable for evaluation of strength, mobility, and co-ordination (see Chap. 7). Usually a ball of 45 or 55 cm is used since this size ball can easily be carried around. Although the ball rolls more easily when the exercises are done on a firm mat, they can also be done in the patient's bed.

9.22 "Perpetual Motion"

Constant location exercise; Fig. 9.22.

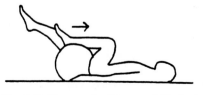

Fig. 9.22. The exercise "Perpetual Motion".

Objectives
- To practice hip flexion and abduction and hip extension and adduction
- To practice hip and knee flexion and extension in good alignment of thigh, lower leg, and foot
- To train alternate leg movement as required in gait
- To test balance, coordination, and the ability to dissociate legs
- To decrease the weight of the leg during flexion and extension
- To strengthen hip and trunk extensor muscles
- To evaluate hip extensor muscle strength
- To train the quadriceps muscle eccentrically
- To move legs alternately at gait velocity

Ball Size. The diameter of the ball should be approximately the length of the thigh.

Starting Position. Supine on the floor, mat, or bed, the left (right) leg rests extended with the calf or the heel on top of the ball, and the right (left) leg is flexed in hip and knee at approximately 90°-90°. The arms are extended and resting with the hands (palms down) near the pelvis.

Actio. There are two simultaneous actios:
- The left (right) leg pulls the ball into flexion of hip and knee and maybe some abduction (and external rotation of the thigh and medial rotation of the knee).
- The right (left) heel pushes upward and forward until the leg (tentacle) extends.

Reactio. There are two simultaneous reactios:
- Mobilization of the left (right) leg into flexion of the hip and the knee (concentric hamstring and hip flexor muscles activity.)
- Mobilization of extension of the right (left) knee, concentric activity of the quadriceps muscle, eccentric activity of the hip flexor muscles and stabilizing activity of the abdominal and trunk extensor muscles.

Return Actio. There are two simultaneous return actios:
- The left (right) leg/heel pushes the ball into extension and slight adduction (medial rotation of the thigh and external rotation of the knee).
- The right (left) leg flexes in knee and hip.

Return Reactio. There are two simultaneous reactios:
- Mobilization of extension of the left (right) hip and knee, eccentric hip flexor and hamstring muscle activity.
- Mobilization of flexion of the right (left) hip and knee, concentric hip flexor muscle activity, eccentric quadriceps muscle activity.

Conditios
- Both legs move in a sagittal plane.
- The ball rolls in a straight line.
- Trunk, head, and arms remain in contact with the floor.
- The right (left) heel should not be lowered below knee level during the return actio.
- There should be no unwanted acceleration of the movement.

Speed. The ideal speed is gait velocity, but in the beginning the patient can move more slowly while learning the movement.

Caution, Notes
- Adaptations may be necessary to observe hip or knee precautions.
- Stabilization can be gained by lifting the pelvis up when the leg on the ball is extended (Fig. 13.20).
- The exercise can be made more difficult by flexing the elbows to decrease the BOS, then lifting the arms at approximately 90° shoulder flexion.
- The exercise can be performed on the PhysioRoll.
- Initially both legs can be placed on the ball to practice bilateral hip flexion and extension.
- The exercise can be used as a starting position for manual therapy on the lower extremities, with the therapist sitting on the ball (see Chap. 8).
- Children under the age of 5 years may have difficulty coordinating the movement of the legs.
- Observation of the movement gives the therapist information about the patient's ability to coordinate the movement of his legs at gait velocity, his ability to dissociate, and the strength of the hip extensor muscles.
- The exercise promotes venous return which benefits patients with lymphedema of the legs.
- Dots can be placed on the distal thigh and the foot to increase awareness for alignment (Fig. 11.6).

Examples
- A patient with Parkinson's disease who begins to have difficulty moving his legs alternately at gait speed.
- A patient who has suffered a stroke and has only mild spasticity and needs to practice selective movements of the hips into flexion and extension.
- The stabilizing variation may benefit a patient suffering from degenerative joint disease of the hips who can master the mobilizing variation and needs strengthening of the hip extensor muscles.

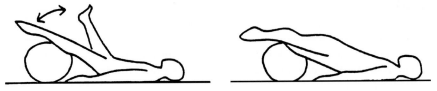

Fig. 9.23. The exercise "Pendulum".

9.23 "Pendulum"

Constant location exercise; Fig. 9.23.

Objectives
- To mobilize the hip ab- and adductor muscles
- To strengthen the hip ab- and adductor muscles in an open and closed kinetic chain
- To strengthen the "rotator cuff" of the pelvic girdle
- To evaluate strength of the hip ab- and adductor muscles
- To train timing and skill of the hip ab- and adductor muscles and rotator cuff muscles of the pelvis
- To strengthen the abdominal muscles
- To strengthen back extensor muscles
- To facilitate rotation of the lower thoracic spine

Ball Size. The same as in the "Perpetual Motion." A slightly larger ball makes it easier to braid one leg under the other.

Starting Position. Supine with the arms extended, slightly abducted, and palms down near the pelvis. The left (right) leg rests with the heel and lower part of the calf on top of the ball. The right (left) leg is flexed at approximately 90° at the hip joint, and the knee is fully extended (unless there is tightness of the hamstring muscles which prevent full extension).

Mobilizing Variation

First Actio. The right (left) leg is the tentacle which moves in a transverse plane to the left (right) side (Fig. 7.10a,b).

First Reactio. The left (right) leg which is positioned on the ball moves with the ball to the right (left) side to maintain the equilibrium.

Second Actio. The right (left) leg moves in a transverse plane to the right (left) side.

Second Reactio. The left (right) leg moves with the ball to the left (right) side to maintain the equilibrium.

Stabilizing Variation

Starting Position. Same as above except for the left (right) leg is positioned closer to the knee on the ball (Figs. 7.13a,b, 11.8).

First Actio. The pelvis lifts off the mat, extending the hips when the right (left) tentacle leg flexes in the hip joint moving in a transverse plane to the left side.

First Reactio. The left (right) leg rolls on the ball on its lateral side controlling the rolling movement of the ball. There is a counterclockwise rotation of the pelvis continuing to the lower thoracic spine. The left (right) hip abductor muscles are in a bridge activity in a closed kinetic chain. The right (left) leg crosses over the left (right) leg, the right (left) hip abductor muscles are in a free-play function in an open kinetic chain. The head, upper trunk, shoulder girdle, and arms stabilize reactively and maintain contact with the floor.

Second Actio. The right (left) tentacle leg moves in a transverse plane to the right; the right (left) knee flexes and braids under the left (right) leg. The pelvis is still lifted, with the left (right) hip extended.

Second Reactio. The left (right) leg rolls on the ball on its medial side controlling the movement of the ball. There is a clockwise rotation of the pelvis continuing to the lower thoracic spine. The left (right) adductor muscles are in a bridge activity in a closed kinetic chain. The right (left) leg is under the left (right) leg flexed in the knee, and the adductor muscles in a open kinetic chain in a free play function. The head, upper trunk, shoulder girdle, and arms stabilize reactively.

Conditios
- The head, shoulder girdle, and arms keep contact with the floor, unless a variation of the exercise is planned.
- During the mobilizing version the pelvis remains in a neutral position on the floor.

Speed. Comfortable speed; there should be no unwanted acceleration when changing directions.

Caution, Notes
- Hip precautions must be observed. A sandbag, towel, or half a foam roll can be placed midline to prevent the ball from rolling into adduction.
- The patient should master the mobilizing version before attempting the stabilizing version.
- The exercise is very difficult if the arms are flexed, put in an asymmetrical position (e.g., one arm placed behind the head), or elevated.
- Tight hamstring muscles require flexion at the knee (not extension at the hip) as adaptation when the leg moves in a transverse plane.

- Both variations give information about the patient's skill, coordination, and timing problems.
- The second variation provides information about strength, mobility, and skill.

Examples
- A patient who after surgery to his leg is allowed to move his non-weight-bearing leg in all planes. Place the weight-bearing leg on the ball and use the non-weight-bearing leg as the pendulum to strengthen it in all planes.
- A patient with multiple sclerosis strengthens and coordinates her legs with the help of the therapist (Fig. 7.10).

The following exercises – "Move My Leg" and "Rock'n Roll" – were developed from the previous two exercises for the benefit of the therapist. I often found myself in need of a therapist after working in intensive care and with tall patients who had substantial spasticity. I also felt that additional arms were needed to manage patients with high muscle tone. I was not tall enough to comfortably lift and move a spastic, paralyzed, or weak leg. These exercises were solutions to my problems.

9.24 "Rock'n Roll"

Constant location exercise; Fig. 9.24.

Objectives
- To facilitate trunk rotation and hip flexion/extension in patients with high tone (spasticity)
- To provide proprioceptive input
- To decrease the amount of weight the weak patient must move or lift
- To allow for passive range of motion of hips and knees into flexion/extension and ab- and adduction

Ball Size. Diameter of the ball should be approximately the length of the therapist's lower leg – larger if the patient has very long legs.

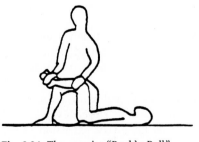

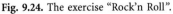

Fig. 9.24. The exercise "Rock'n Roll".

Starting Position. The patient is supine on the floor or a mat table, legs in approximately 90° hip, and knee flexion. The therapist sits on a ball at approximately the level of the patient's hips, one of her legs placed alongside the trunk and the other under the patient's lower legs (see Fig. 8.13).

Actio. The therapist moves the ball with her own legs in the desired direction so that the patient's legs move into flexion/extension or ab- and adduction or rotation of the pelvis.

Reactio. The therapist has her hands free to stroke, tap, distract/compress the joints or use the hands for stabilization while moving the patient's legs and pelvis. This can lead to decreased muscle tone in a spastic patient (Fig. 13.19).

Conditio
• The patient's trunk remains in contact with the floor/mat.

Speed. Slow and rhythmic, rocking and rolling.

Caution, Notes
• Observe precautions.
• Movements can be performed with one or both legs in a pattern of proprioceptive neuromuscular facilitation (see Fig. 8.13).
• The position can be used for manual therapy of the lower extremity (see Figs. 8.14–8.16).
• The therapist can sit on the ball between the flexed legs and gently bounce/rock the pelvis.

Examples
• Patients with severe muscle tone flexor or extensor pattern after a stroke or multiple sclerosis.
• When performing manual therapy (see Chap. 8).

9.25 "Move My Leg"

Constant location exercise; Fig. 9.25.

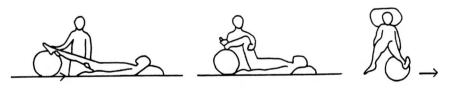

Fig. 9.25. The exercise "Move My Legs".

Objectives
- To ease the range of motion exercises for bedridden or weak patients (Fig. 11.3)
- To enable the patient to see his leg for feedback with trace or no movement patients (Fig. 7.21)
- To enable the therapist or family to be able to move the leg without having to lift it (Figs. 7.21, 10.1a,b, 10.3c, 10.4c)
- To promote venous return in patients with edema/swelling of their leg or legs (Fig. 11.1a)

Ball Size. A diameter of 45 or 55 cm is usually sufficient.

Starting Position. Supine position, one or both legs placed on the ball.

Actio. Depends on the goal and the strength of the patient. The therapist/family can actively assist with the range of motion; the weak patient can move his leg without having to lift it. The movement direction can be flexion/extension of hip and knees or ab- and adduction of the hips.

Reactio. Depends on the patient's condition and the goal and direction of the movement.

Conditio. The movement of the leg should be assisted by the therapist/family so that the leg does not "fall" off the ball.

Speed. Slow enough for the patient to see the movement.

Caution, Other
- Dots can be placed on foot and knee to increase the patient's awareness (Fig. 7.21).
- The movements can be actively assisted (Fig. 10.3).
- For patients with mild spasticity the exercise can help to promote selective movements.
- Weak patients find it helpful to place the ball behind the knees when stretching their hamstrings (Figs. 7.4c, 10.6a,b).
- When sitting at the edge of bed or in a chair, the patient can place the ball on the floor to perform active range of motion of the ankles (Fig. 7.20c).

Examples
- Patient in intensive care and those who need assistance when weak or paralyzed (Figs. 7.6, 10.3).

The "Easter Bunny" and "Well Figure" are Klein-Vogelbach exercises for promoting reactive hip extension.

9.26 "Easter Bunny"

Constant location exercise; Fig. 9.26.

Objectives
- To mobilize hip extension in an unstable position
- To mobilize hip extension as typical in gait
- To practice eccentric and concentric quadriceps training
- To promote good postural alignment of the trunk and pelvis during forward movement

Ball Size. The diameter of the ball is approximately the length of the patient's thigh.

Starting Position. The patient kneels behind the ball on the right (left) knee with the hip slightly flexed. The left (right) leg rests on top of the ball. The trunk is aligned and leans slightly backward. The toes of the right (left) foot are extended and placed in a sagittal plane behind the left (right) hip joint. The arms form an oval in a transverse plane at shoulder level.

Actio. The right (left) foot pushes off with the toes into pronation of the forefoot, knee, and hip extension.

Reactio. The ball and body are accelerated and moved forward. The right (left) leg is in a bridge activity, the left (right) foot reaches the floor, and the leg is flexed and slightly externally rotated. The right (left) hip extends from the distal lever. Because of the right (left) foot's position there is a slight internal rotation of the right (left) leg in the hip joint.

Conditios
- The pelvis remains in the frontal plane throughout the movement.
- The trunk remains aligned but may lean slightly forward to avoid hyperextension of the lumbar spine.

Speed. Comfortable speed, depending on the strength of the patient's leg which is pushing off. There should be no uncontrolled acceleration.

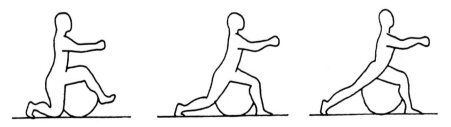

Fig. 9.26. The exercise "Easter Bunny".

Caution, Notes

- Since the trunk leans slightly backward when starting, the quadriceps is loaded eccentrically.
- Returning slowly to the starting position requires substantial eccentric quadriceps activity of the right (left) leg.
- The exercise can be practiced between two chairs. Stabilizing the shoulder girdle on chairs makes it easier to learn the exercise.
- To make the exercise easier, choose a smaller ball and let the left (right) foot rest on the floor during the forward movement.
- To make the exercise more difficult, the heel of the anterior leg can be lifted to decrease the BOS.
- A heavy wide pelvis makes balancing more difficult for the patient. Practicing (between chairs) may be necessary.
- A long trunk and heavy arms make balancing more difficult. Allowing the hands to be placed on the ball may help stabilize trunk and arms.
- Padding may be put under the knee if it is sensitive (or a Sitfit to increase the challenge).
- The exercise can initially be practiced on a smaller PhysioRoll to make it easier.
- In the end position the patient can activate his pelvic floor muscles by pulling the ischial tuberosities toward the knee, which is in front of the ball, and a spatially fixed point.

Examples

- Patients with sports injuries of the lower extremities who need retraining of skill and strength of the quadriceps muscle
- Patients with poor hip extension who require retraining of postural alignment of the trunk.
- Patients with weak pelvic floor muscles (Figs. 11.30 a,b).

9.27 "Well Figure"

Constant location exercise; Fig. 9.27.

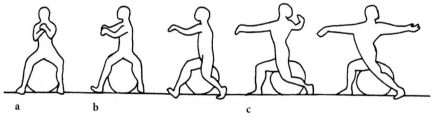

Fig. 9.27 a–c. The exercise "Well Figure".

Objectives
- To mobilize hip extension
- To achieve hip extension from the distal lever as typical in gait
- To practice rotation of the trunk and pelvis on a stable leg

Ball Size. Same diameter as in the "Cowboy," that is, slightly more than the distance from the knee to the floor.

Starting Position. The exercise has three phases. In the starting position the patient sits on the ball, as in the "Cowboy" but with the feet wide apart. The knees and feet point forward. The arms are flexed, with the hands placed on the sternum.

Phase I (Fig. 9.27 a)

First Actio. The initial movement comes from the upper extremities. The arms extend forward in a transverse plane.

First Reactio. In the bridge formed by the legs and the ball, the ball rolls straight backward, resulting in some knee extension and plantar flexion of the feet.

Phase II (Fig. 9.27 b)

Second Actio. The primary movement is in the trunk (tentacle). The stabilized trunk rotates clockwise (counterclockwise) taking the arms along until they form a horizontal oval above the right (left) thigh.

Second Reactio. The left (right) anterior superior iliac spine moves horizontally in a clockwise (counterclockwise) direction. While the right (left) foot turns clockwise (counterclockwise) on the heel, the left (right) toe turns the same direction on the toes. The ball also rolls clockwise (counterclockwise) with a little twist. The left (right) knee moves medially and downward while the body–ball contact changes. Now only the dorsal/lateral side of the right (left) thigh/buttock is touching the ball.

Phase III (Fig. 9.27 c)

Third Actio. The primary movement is in the tentacle. The right (left) arm continues to move clockwise (counterclockwise) in the transverse plane of the shoulder girdle. The left (right) arm moves counterclockwise (clockwise) in the same plane until both arms are at the side of the trunk with the right (left) palm facing upward and the left (right) palm facing downward. The head continues to rotate clockwise (counterclockwise).

Third Reactio. The ball rolls toward the right (left) heel. The left (right) heel extends toward the floor. The left (right) knee extends. The weight bearing of the lower extremities changes from a parking position to a support activity. The left (right) quadriceps muscle is in a bridge activity. The hamstring muscles of the right (left) leg must stabilize the ball and pull it forward.

Conditios
- During the first two phases the legs remain parked.
- The distances between sternal notch and xiphoid process and navel do not change.
- The pelvis remains in a frontal plane during the third phase and is at a right angle to the direction of movement.

Speed. Comfortable speed so the patient can learn each phase of the exercise.

Caution, Notes
- Parts of the exercise can be prepracticed on a stool.
- Each phase of the exercise can be practiced separately.
- The legs should be in good alignment.
- The trunk should remain in good alignment throughout the exercise.
- The last phase of the exercise can be used to strengthen the pelvic floor muscles if the patient is instructed to pull the ischial tuberosities toward the leg, which is in front of the ball, and to use the knees as spatially fixed points.

Examples. As previous exercise.

The following two exercises are favorite exercises of patients with weaknesses of the lower extremities, and patients who need vastus medialis training, open/closed kinetic chain exercises and proper weight bearing.

9.28 "Cocktail Party"

Either constant or changing location exercise; Fig. 9.28.

Objectives
- To achieve automatic weight bearing on one leg in a closed kinetic chain

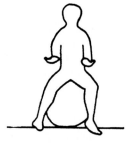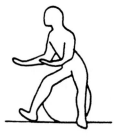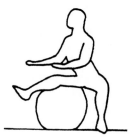

Fig. 9.28. The exercise "Cocktail Party".

- To train the vastus medialis of the quadriceps muscle in a closed kinetic chain
- To stretch the hamstring muscles by strengthening the quadriceps muscle in an open kinetic chain
- To change from an open to a closed kinetic chain for lower extremity strengthening
- To train skill and coordination of lower extremity muscles while stabilizing the trunk

Ball Size. The size of the ball is the same as in the "Cowboy." A larger ball is necessary if the patient does not have full range of motion of the knees or hips. The patient should be able to sit erect on the ball.

Starting Position. The same as in the "Cowboy," except that the legs are slightly more abducted, feet and knees pointing forward. The arms are elevated and flexed in the elbows, palms up as if holding a tray. The head, trunk, and arms are the tentacle.

Actio. The primary movement is in the tentacle. The trunk leans forward and to the right (left), while the left (right) foot turns on the toes moving the left (right) heel to the left (right).

Reactio. The ball moves in a diagonal direction behind the left (right) leg. The right (left) leg loses contact with the floor. The right (left) lower leg extends reactively to counterbalance the weight of the trunk. The right (left) quadriceps muscle is activated reactively in an open kinetic chain, stretching the hamstring muscles of the same leg. The quadriceps muscle of the left (right) leg stabilizes the left (right) leg. The vastus medialis of the left (right) quadriceps muscle is aligned and activated. The left (right) buttock loses contact with the ball (Fig. 6.3).

Conditios
- The distance between symphysis pubis and sternal notch remains the same.
- The leg which is in a closed kinetic chain must be well aligned.
- The forearms remain horizontal in space at all times.

Speed. Slow at first, until the patient knows the exercise. Ideally the tentacle moves approximately 40 times per minute forward/backward.

Caution, Notes
- The patient should be allowed to bear weight on both legs.
- The exercise can be prepracticed between two chairs.
- Use a firm ball when the patient is heavy or needs more challenge.
- Use a softer ball for patients with wide hips.

- The exercise can be done with changing location. The patient then starts with the feet closer together. During the actio the patient pushes off with the left (right) leg, and takes two steps backward in a diagonal direction. The first step to the left (right) side; the second step is backward, changing from weight bearing on two legs to one-legged weight bearing on the left leg only. In the end position the right (left) leg rests on top of the ball. Skill, coordination, and timing is required.

Examples
- Patients 3–6 weeks after anterior cruciate ligament reconstruction to retrain strength, skill and coordination of the lower extremity muscles (Figs. 11.7, 11.9).
- Child with postural deficits learns to lean the stable trunk forward while weight bearing on the legs (this prepares the child for doing the "Cocktail Party" later; Fig. 11.21g)
- As a progression of the "Scale" exercise.

9.29 "Dolphin"

Either constant or location changing exercise; Fig. 9.29.

Objectives
- To practice reactive steps from side to side
- To train alternate weight bearing
- To practice arm swing in the frontal plane
- To train automatic alignment of the lower extremities

Ball Size. The same as the "Cowboy," with a diameter roughly half the length of the leg. Patients with long thighs need a larger ball. The ball should be firm.

Starting Position. Sitting on the ball as in the "Cowboy." The left (right) arm is lifted above the head in a midfrontal plane, the palm pointing toward the head. The right (left) hand rests in the midfrontal plane palm down on the ball.

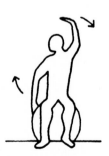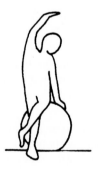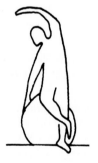

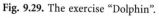

Fig. 9.29. The exercise "Dolphin".

Actio. The actio is initiated by the left (right) arm falling in a semicircular movement in the midfrontal plane. To increase the action, the right (left) arm is raised in the same plane in a semicircular movement at the same time.

Reactio. The ball rolls in a straight line to the right, the movement is accelerated by raising the right (left) arm. The right (left) ischial tuberosity loses contact with the ball, and the right (left) leg takes a reactive step to find a new BOS. The left (right) leg loses contact with the floor and crosses in front of the right (left) leg. The left (right) hand rests on the ball, the right (left) arm is above the head in the midfrontal plane.

Conditios
- The arms move in the midfrontal plane.
- The ball rolls in a straight line from side to side.
- The foot, lower leg, and thigh must be aligned.

Speed. Comfortable speed at first, faster when the patient has mastered the skill. Ideally, approximately 40 rolls per minute.

Caution, Other
- The patient must be able to bear weight on both legs.
- The patient can practice the sideways movement of the feet first by taking approximately five quick alternate steps to one side and then to the other side.
- The hand on the ball controls the ball movement.
- Patients with a heavy wide pelvis have more difficulty getting on one leg when the pelvis loses contact with the ball.
- To perform the location-changing variation, the size of the steps from side to side increases, and the patient loses contact with the ball except for the hand opposite to the weight-bearing leg.

Examples
- Patients functioning at a high level who recover from sport injuries of the lower extremities.
- Patients with difficulty doing alternate weight bearing on the lower extremities e.g., after sports injuries (Fig. 11.14).

Therapists should remember that there are many more ways to use the Swiss ball to treat or retrain patients. The following chapters supply clinical examples.

9.30 Summary of Exercises

Exercises Stabilizing the Spine
- 9.1 Cowboy
- 9.2 Scale
- 9.3 Indian Fakir

- 9.7   Hula-Hula, Forward/Backward (thoracic spine)
- 9.8   Hula-Hula, Side to Side (thoracic spine)
- 9.10 Swing
- 9.13 Trot (rotation)
- 9.16 Walking on Hands
- 9.18 Figurehead
- 9.19 Scissors
- 9.21 Carrousel
- 9.26 Easter Bunny
- 9.27 Well Figure
- 9.28 Cocktail Party

Exercises Mobilizing the Spine
- 9.4   Donkey Stretch Yourself (flexion/extension)
- 9.6   Sea Gull (extension)
- 9.7   Hula-Hula, Forward/Backward (flexion/extension of the lumbar spine)
- 9.8   Hula-Hula, Side to Side (lateral flexion of the lumbar spine)
- 9.9   Salamander (lateral flexion)
- 9.11 Duck (extension of the lumbar spine)
- 9.14 Sea Urchin (flexion)
- 9.15 Goldfish (extension)
- 9.18 Figurehead (extension)
- 9.19 Scissors (rotation)
- 9.20 Mermaid (lateral flexion)
- 9.27 Well Figure (rotation)
- 9.29 Dolphin (lateral flexion)

Exercises for Postural Training
- 9.1   Cowboy
- 9.2   Scale
- 9.3   Indian Fakir
- 9.7   Hula-Hula, Forward/Backward
- 9.8   Hula-Hula, Side to Side
- 9.21 Carrousel
- 9.26 Easter Bunny
- 9.27 Well Figure
- 9.28 Cocktail Party

Exercises for Abdominal Training
- 9.1   Cowboy
- 9.2   Scale
- 9.3   Indian Fakir
- 9.14 Sea Urchin
- 9.16 Walking on Hands
- 9.22 Perpetual Motion
- 9.23 Pendulum

Exercises Adaptable for Pelvic Floor Muscle Training (see also Chap. 14)
- 9.1 Cowboy
- 9.2 Scale
- 9.7 Hula-Hula Forward/Backward
- 9.8 Hula-Hula Side to Side
- 9.11 Duck
- 9.26 Easter Bunny
- 9.27 Well Figure

Exercises for Back Extensor Training
- 9.1 Cowboy
- 9.2 Scale
- 9.3 Indian Fakir
- 9.21 Carrousel
- 9.22 Perpetual Motion
- 9.23 Pendulum

Exercising for Strengthening and Mobilizing the Shoulder
- 9.15 Goldfish
- 9.14 Sea Urchin (Drunken Sea Urchin, for horizontal ab- and adduction of the shoulder from the proximal lever)
- 9.16 Walking on Hands
- 9.17 Push Me–Pull Me
- 9.19 Scissors (horizontal ab- and adduction of the shoulder from the proximal lever)
- 9.10 Swing
- 9.12 Crab
- 9.13 Trot
- 9.9 Salamander (all the above exercises are in closed chain activity or support function)
- 9.18 Figurehead (and Scale and Dolphin are open kinetic chain activity or play function)
- 9.2 Scale (variation with arm movements)
- 9.29 Dolphin

Exercises for Mobilizing and Stabilizing the Hips
- 9.2 Scale
- 9.3 Indian Fakir
- 9.4 Donkey Stretch Yourself
- 9.5 Stretch Myself
- 9.7 Hula-Hula, Forward/Backward
- 9.8 Hula-Hula, Side to Side
- 9.14 Sea Urchin
- 9.15 Goldfish
- 9.22 Perpetual Motion
- 9.23 Pendulum
- 9.27 Well Figure

Exercises for Pregait Training
- 9.1 Cowboy
- 9.2 Scale
- 9.3 Indian Fakir
- 9.4 Donkey Stretch Yourself
- 9.22 Perpetual Motion
- 9.26 Easter Bunny
- 9.27 Well Figure

Exercises for Alignment of the Lower Extremities
- 9.1 Cowboy
- 9.2 Scale
- 9.3 Indian Fakir
- 9.4 Donkey Stretch Yourself
- 9.5 Stretch Myself
- 9.7 Hula-Hula, Forward/Backward
- 9.22 Perpetual Motion
- 9.28 Cocktail Party
- 9.29 Dolphin

Exercises for Reactive Steps
- 9.3 Indian Fakir
- 9.4 Donkey Stretch Yourself
- 9.21 Carrousel
- 9.28 Cocktail Party
- 9.29 Dolphin

References

Carrière B (1993) Swiss ball exercises. PT Magazine Phys Ther 9:92–100

Kenneally M, Rubenach H, Elvey R (1988) Assessment of abnormal movement patterns in musculoskeletal disorders. In: Grant R (ed) Physical therapy of the cervical and thoracic spine. Churchill Livingstone, New York, pp 167–194

Klein-Vogelbach S (1990a) Ballgymnastik zur Funktionellen Bewegungslehre, 3rd edn. Springer, Berlin Heidelberg New York

Klein-Vogelbach S (1990b) Functional kinetics. Springer, Berlin Heidelberg New York

Klein-Vogelbach S (1990c) Functional kinetics: Swiss ball videotape. Springer, Berlin Heidelberg New York

10 Intensive and Acute Care

OBJECTIVES

By the end of this chapter the reader will be able to:
- Understand the purpose of using the Swiss ball in intensive and acute care
- Know the precautions for the Swiss ball in intensive care
- Select patients who may benefit from the Swiss ball
- Instruct the family in performing exercises with the patient

10.1 Introduction

Intensive and acute care is an area that is often neglected in physical therapy. Especially those who are still new in the profession often feel ill-prepared for work in an environment that is so dominated by intimidating machines and alarms and a general atmosphere of anxiety. Many others may prefer to avoid this environment because they have no prior experience, lack ideas or imagination concerning goals, or are simply fearful. Young physical therapists are in need of new and stimulating ideas to guide them through the maze of intensive and acute care.

Physical therapy in intensive and acute care has changed tremendously over the years. Physicians now ask physical therapists to evaluate the patient and provide input instead of merely giving them orders for range of motion (ROM) or to sit a patient. Nowadays physical therapists actively help in managing the critically ill patient and are members of the team of physicians, nurses, respiratory therapists, and family who begin on day 1 to rehabilitate the patient, regardless of whether he is on a respirator, in a comatose state, or recovering from surgery. It is important to remember that exercises can encourage patient participation while the therapist maintains a level of assistance that prevents abnormal tone or tonus overcompensation for the desired activity.

> The role of the physical therapist, like of every member of the health care team, is to help the patient regain homeostasis.

The way in which this is accomplished may be dramatically affected by decisions made by the physical therapist. In intensive and acute care the physical therapist spends more continuous time (often 30–45 minutes daily) working with the patient than any other member of the team.

Physical therapists become involved with the patient before speech and occupational therapists, and they work closely with nurses and respiratory therapists, unless they are performing chest physical therapy themselves (Carrière 1993).

> The patient's length of stay in the hospital may depend on early physical therapy intervention in critical care (Welch and Anastasas 1996).

Progress in the recovery (e.g., a comatose patient waking up, return of muscle function) is frequently noticed first by therapists and is often attributed to the early intervention. Physical therapists are helpful in recognizing early signs of complications (e.g., deep vein thrombosis, heterotopic ossification) and can therefore provide important information to the physician and nurses. They are also able to instruct the family and nurses in the correct positioning of the patient. The therapists also teach the family how to exercise the patient as well as help them understand the recovery process (Carrière 1993).

> Especially with patients in a comatose state the therapists and family must overcome their own fears and establish a dialogue with them. The responses to treatment that these patients show may be very subtle, such as a change in respiratory or heart rate or a motor response such as smacking the lips, chewing motion, change in the facial expression, or *flexion/extension synergies* (Ziegler 1996).

The *Glasgow Coma Scale* (Teasdale and Jennett 1974; Jennett and Teasdale 1981) was developed to assess the depth and duration of impaired consciousness and coma and helps the therapist in evaluating the patient to recognize changes. The Glasgow Coma Scale evaluates eye opening and best motor and verbal responses. The highest score is 15, when a patient can open the eyes spontaneously, obeys motor commands, and is oriented.

Physical therapy treatment has changed in keeping with new understanding of neurophysiology and physiology (see Chap. 2) and of motor learning (see Chap. 3). Davies (1994) integrates new treatment approaches to provide innovative ideas about early rehabilitation after traumatic brain injuries and severe brain lesions. Many other recent publications help therapists working in hospitals. For example, Mauritz (1994) describes rehabilitation after a stroke and includes the early phase of treatment, Buck and Beckers (1993) deal with rehabilitation of spinal cord injuries, and Umphred (1995) provides a wonderful resource for understanding the medical problems of a neurological patient.

Countless articles and papers offer the therapist help in facing problems with patients in intensive and acute care. The *Journal of the American Physical Therapy Association* devoted the May and June of 1996 issues to cardiopulmonary physical therapy. This special series includes an excellent review about cardiac transplant by Sadowsky (1996), and a contribution by Ciccone (1996) on current trends in cardiovascular pharmacology which can help the therapist understand the medication given to patients and its effects on them. Peel (1996) describes the cardiopulmonary system and movement dysfunction and helps the therapist to recognize signs of respiratory distress, inadequate cardiac output, etc. Cahalin (1996) reviews heart failure and the benefits of treatment. In an article on outcomes in cardiopulmonary rehabilitation Pashkow (1996) reviews outcome data which support the view that exercising benefits patients suffering from cardiopulmonary dysfunctions. Downs (1996) reviews physical therapy in lung transplantation. Cooper (1995) writes about exercises for patients with chronic pulmonary disease. All these articles can assist the therapist dealing with acutely ill patients.

> The exercise program for patients with bone marrow transplant should be designed to reduce the effects of immobility and prolonged bed rest and as to maintain the level of cardiopulmonary endurance and muscle strength (Sayre and Marcoux 1992; Adams 1995).

Simionato et al. (1988) describe neural tension signs in patients with Guillain-Barré syndrome and stress the importance of careful attention to the patient's symptoms and signs during assessment and treatment. Clinical examples and case reports such as this help the therapist to understand the many problems encountered in critical and acute care.

The least problematic patients are those receiving total hip and knee replacements, provided that there are no additional medical problems.

After consulting with the physician or the team involved (especially nurses and respiratory therapists) the physical therapist evaluates the patient, draws conclusions, and then begins treatment. The following are examples of how to use the Swiss ball, the precautions to be observed, and how to select and apply exercises to the patient.

10.2 Applications

The Swiss ball can be used in critical and acute care for:
- Passive/active assistance of ROM
- Strengthening/stretching
- Cardiopulmonary training
- Mobilization of neural structures

- Management of muscle tonus
- Positioning
- Family training

Precautions
- Keep the Swiss ball clean.
- Try not to place the ball on the floor, and wash it before using it. If possible, supply the patient with his own ball.
- Watch for lines, tubes, and monitors

Preparation of the Patient/Family

> Talking to the patient and family prepares them for the planned activity. This may decrease the anxiety level of the patient, who is already in a stressful environment. It is also important to talk to a comatose patient, who may be unable to react but may still hear and feel.

If the family understands why and how the exercises are performed, they become an ally and can help the therapist. Patient, family, and therapist should have a common goal.

10.3 Selection of Patients

The Swiss ball can be used by all physical therapy disciplines, especially when patients are very weak and heavy.

10.3.1 Neurology

In neurological patients the ball can be used for positioning, ROM, decreasing the weight of the paralyzed limb, management of tonus, and mobilizing neural structures.

EXAMPLES

Figure 10.1. An 11-year-old child suffering from respiratory arrest after a status asthmaticus is in a comatose state (Glasgow Coma Scale 4–5) with decerebrate posturing. The patient reacted to pain and had no verbal responses.

Panels a, b. After being instructed by the physical therapist 9 days after the respiratory arrest, the father of the child is doing ROM of the lower extremities with the Swiss ball, including gentle mobilization of trunk rotation (a), flexion/extension of the legs, and hip ab- and adduction (b).

Panels c, d. Four days later the patient is extubated and begins sitting with the help of the father and the physical therapist (frequently therapy is initiated earlier, and if stable, sitting begins as shown in the pictures). The Swiss ball is used to position the child in an upright sitting position, mobilize the spine gently into extension (c), begin weight bearing of the upper extremities, mobilize the shoulder/arms, and work on trunk elongation (d). The father continues to do ROM with the child two or three times a day and on weekends. According to the family, less than 1 year later the child had fully recovered.

Figure 10.2. An approximately 40-year old patient spent about 6 months in intensive care on a respirator following a severe case of Guillain-Barré syndrome. In addition to using the Swiss ball for ROM of the lower extremities into flexion/extension of ankle, knee, and hip and ab- and adduction of the hip, it is also used to mobilize the spine. The example shows the patient 104 and 153 days after onset of the disease. The patient is still unable to actively move his legs. He suffers from considerable pain and has limited tolerance to exercises. He enjoys sitting and actively mobilizing the spine (a–e) and is able to move the arms actively in flexion and extension when the weight of the arms is resting on a Swiss ball (f, g). The wrists are supported by a splint to avoid overstretching.

Figure 10.3. A 43-year-old patient who suffered a stroke resulting in paralysis of the left side begins in intensive care with Swiss ball exercises. Dots are placed on the hand, knee, and foot to increase the awareness of the left side and to stimulate visual tracts while the movement is done passively by the physical therapist (a, b). When the leg is elevated on the Swiss ball, the weight of the leg is reduced, and the patient can observe the movement (c).

In patients with hemiplegia the strength of the abdominal muscles is important for the stability of the trunk as a solid base for the shoulder/scapula muscles (Klein-Vogelbach 1963; Davies 1990). Therefore early stimulation of the abdominal muscles can also be achieved by moving the head and arms diagonally to the side "unaffected" by the stroke (b).

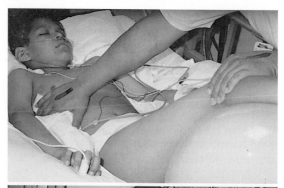

a

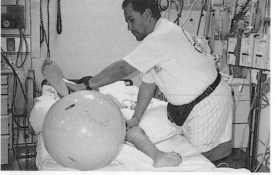

b

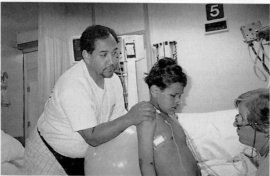

c

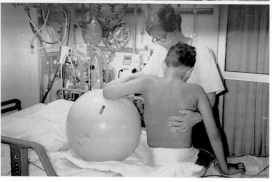

d

Fig. 10.1 a–d. An 11-year-old child in a comatose state. **a.** The child receives mobilization of trunk rotation; the legs are supported on the Swiss ball. **b.** The child's father moves the legs into abduction and adduction of the hips. **c.** The patient sits at the edge of the bed with the trunk supported by the Swiss ball and gently mobilized into extension of the spine. **d.** The Swiss ball placed under the arm helps with elongation of the trunk and mobilization of the left shoulder.

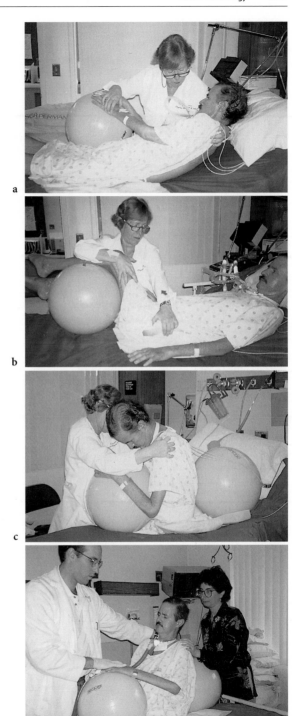

Fig. 10.2 a. The Swiss ball is used to mobilize the spine of this patient with Guillain-Barré syndrome 104 and 153 days after onset into rotation from the upper trunk/ shoulder girdle. **b.** Mobilization of the lower trunk and hips. **c.** Mobilization while sitting into flexion and extension of the spine. **d.** Sitting with the arms supported on a second ball. **e.** Rotation and lateral flexion of the spine in sitting are practiced in combination. **f,g.** After 153 days following the onset of the disease the patient in Fig. 10.3 is able to move his shoulders actively into flexion and extension while supported by the Swiss ball.

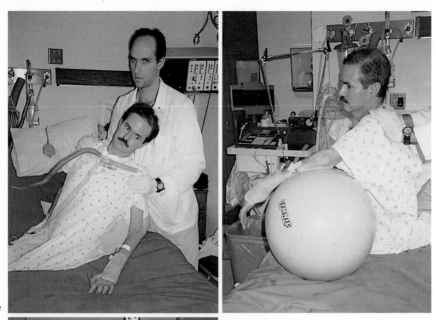

e   f

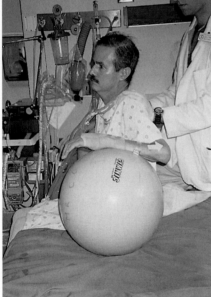

g

Fig. 10.2 e–g.

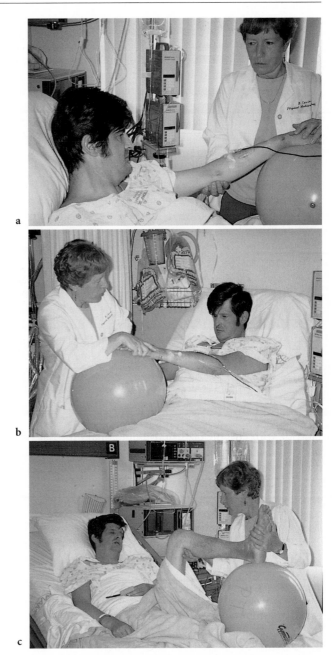

Fig. 10.3 a. A stroke patient observes the movement of his paralyzed arm. **b.** Moving the paralyzed arm diagonally across the body while lifting the head may activate the weakened abdominal muscles. **c.** The patient can observe the movement of the paralyzed leg when it is placed on a Swiss ball.

10.3.2 Cardiology

EXAMPLES

Figure 10.4. A 76-year-old patient was still on a respirator 6 weeks after a myocard infarct and open heart surgery. The patient had an extremely complicated recovery and was very weak and "stiff" from being unable to move. The patient began to open her eyes when sitting, and her muscle tonus improved as well. The patient's daughter and husband exercised daily with the patient using the Swiss ball, the daughter exclaiming, "This saves my back."

Panels a, b. When sitting the patient at the edge of the bed the ball is used either to support the patient's back (a) and gently mobilize it into extension or to position one of her arms (b) to achieve abduction of the shoulder while the wrist with multiple lines rests on the ball.

Panel c. The patient's husband moves her left ankle into dorsiflexion using the Swiss ball.

A patient after a heart transplant with profound weakness from the prolonged hospital stay before the surgery while waiting for a donor. The Swiss ball reduces the weight of the limbs when the patient is actively exercising while waiting for the transplant, and when recovering from the surgery.

10.3.3 Medical/Surgical

Patients with chronic obstructive pulmonary disease often depend at least temporarily on the ventilator. In weaning the patient from the respirator it may be important for him to engage in exercises. The exercises cannot be strenuous but should be active. Casaburi et al. (1991) provide a physiological rational for exercise training of patients with chronic obstructive pulmonary disease.

> **!** **Exercises may remove the acid stimulus to breathing and thereby lower the ventilatory requirements.**

The Swiss ball can enable the patient to exercise without straining himself by reducing the weight of the limbs while exercising. Exercises can be performed with active assistance, as demonstrated in Fig. 10.3c, or actively, as demonstrated in Figs. 10.2f and 10.10g.

Patients with leukemia often spend months in isolation, sometimes in intensive care units. Physical therapy exercise programs must be designed to reduce the effects of immobility and prolonged bed rest and to increase or maintain the current levels of cardiopulmonary endurance and muscle strength (Sayre and Marcoux 1992). Energy conservation is another impor-

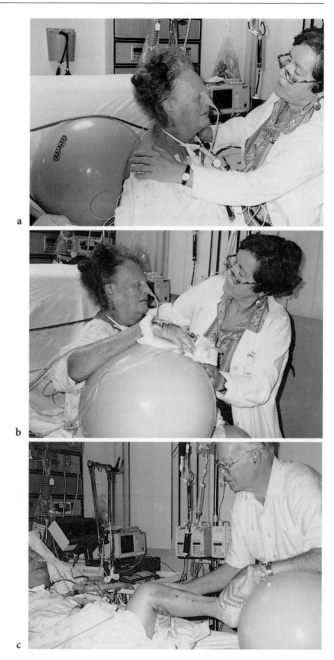

Fig. 10.4 a. The Swiss ball is used to support a cardiac patient while sitting up after a complicated recovery. **b.** The Swiss ball supports and elevates the arm with multiple lines attached to improve ROM of the shoulder. **c.** The patient's husband assists with ROM of the left ankle into dorsiflexion.

tant aspect because the patient's condition may change frequently when he is recovering from the bone marrow transplant and after chemotherapy (Adam 1995). Examples are presented below of the way in which to use the Swiss ball with patients who have received bone marrow transplants and/or chemotherapy. Of course, good hygiene is of the utmost importance. It is a good idea to supply the patient with a new ball, which stays in the patient's room at all times and is cleaned before each treatment session.

EXAMPLES

Figure 10.5. A 5-year-old girl with leukemia and chemotherapy for treatment of the disease suffered from pneumonia and respiratory failure and requires intubation. After the patient was extubated physical therapy in intensive care began for strengthening and mobilizing this very weak patient. The patient's muscle strength was grossly in the fair (3/5) range, she could ambulate only with external support, and she had low endurance.

The Swiss ball serves as a tool which can help make otherwise unpleasant therapy fun and playful. The ball is used in the hospital bed to sit or lie on, to kick, to throw and to "exercise" the patient's favorite toy pet.

Panel a. The child exercises her toy pet while strengthening her legs and mobilizing shoulders and trunk.

Panels b, c. Weight shifting and lifting the ball above her head (and throwing it afterwards to her mother; b) the patient strengthens her right leg by standing on one leg).

Panel d. Both legs are strengthened, and the back and arms are mobilized as the patient pushes away from her feet. The patient also sat on the ball and bounced to obtain proprioceptive input and stimulation of afferences to the central nervous system.

Figure 10.6. A 35-year-old man received an allogenic bone marrow transplant and developed graft-versus-host disease requiring abdominal surgery about 60 days after the transplant. He was very weak (fair muscle strength), had low endurance, and tired after 5 repetitions of exercises. He was able to sit up in a chair for 1 hour on a good day. The patient was attached to multiple lines and remained in isolation. Prior to admission the patient enjoyed exercising and was very athletic. Therapy did not begin until 5 days after the abdominal surgery in order not to strain the abdominal wall.

Panel a. Initial exercises with the Swiss ball allowed the patient to stretch his hamstring and strengthen his quadriceps muscles without straining the abdomen.

Panels b–d. After spending several more months in the hospital he performs exercises with the ball which stretch the entire posterior chain and mobilize the trunk and upper extremities in extension and rotation. Finally, the patient is allowed to leave his room and come to the gymnastic room to use equipment such as a stationary bicycle, and treadmill to rebuild his strength.

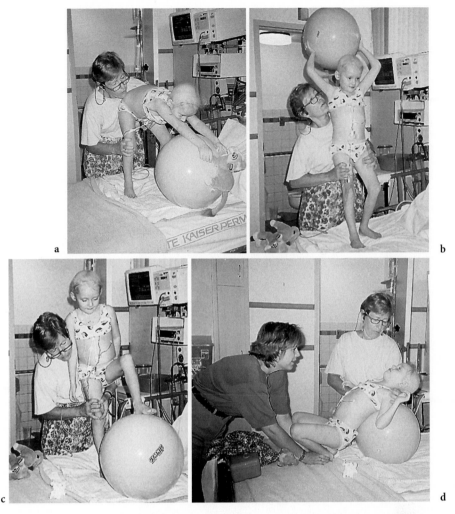

Fig. 10.5a–d. A 5-year-old child suffering from leukemia playfully strengthens and mobilizes her trunk and extremities with the Swiss ball.

The critical care and acute care units present the therapist with numerous possibilities for using the Swiss ball to help manage the very ill patient and allow for a slow progression to increase weight bearing and early active movement. Use of the Swiss ball does not exclude conventional exercising or helping the patient progress to resistive exercises. Often resistance is given while exercising with the Swiss ball. Once the patient is well enough to use the gymnastic room, many of the exercises described in Chap. 9 can be performed.

The following chapters present examples for patients using physical therapy on an out patient basis.

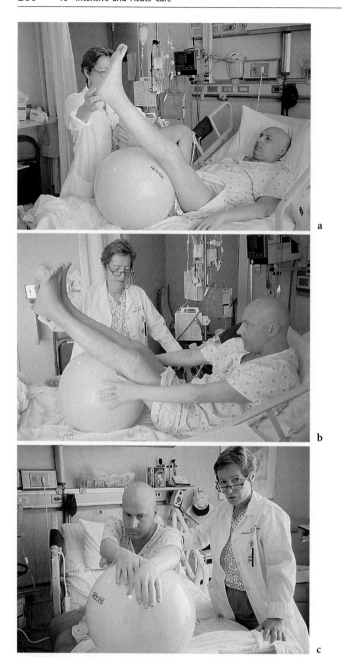

Fig. 10.6a–c. A patient suffering from leukemia. **a.** Seven days after abdominal surgery he begins stretching his hamstrings without straining the abdominal wall. **b.** The patient stretches the posterior chain flexing the head, trunk, and hip extending the knee (and adding dorsiflexion of the foot) using the Swiss ball to support his legs. **c.** The arms are supported on the ball while the patient performs trunk rotation while sitting on the edge of the bed.

References

Adams RC (1995) Bone marrow transplants. Adv Phys Ther 6(44):20, 21, 25

Buck M, Beckers D (1993) Rehabilitation bei Querschnittlähmungen. Springer, Berlin Heidelberg New York

Cahalin LP (1996) Heart failure. Phys Ther 76:516–533

Carrière B (1993) Die Rolle der Krankengymnasten im Team der Neurotraumatologie. Krankengymnastik 7:820–827

Casaburi R, Patessio A, Ioli F, Zanaboni S, Donner CF, Wasserman K (1991) Reduction in exercise lactic acidosis and ventilation as a result of exercise training in patients with obstructive lung disease. Am Rev Respir Dis 143:9–18

Ciccone CD (1996) Current trends in cardiovascular pharmacology. Phys Ther 76:481–497

Cooper CB (1995) Determining the role of exercises in patients with chronic pulmonary disease. Medicine and science in sports and exercise. J Am Coll Sports Med, June:147–157

Davies PM (1990) Right in the middle. Springer, Berlin Heidelberg New York

Davies PM (1994) Starting again. Springer, Berlin Heidelberg New York

Downs AM (1996) Physical therapy in lung transplantation Phys Ther 76:626–642

Jennett B, Teasdale G (1981) Management of head injuries. Davis, Philadelphia

Klein-Vogelbach S (1963) Die Stabilisation der Körpermitte und die aktive Widerlagerbildung als Ausgangspunkt einer Bewegungserziehung (unter besonderer Berücksichtigung der Probleme des Hemiplegikers). Krankengymnastik 5:1–9

Mauritz K-H (1994) Rehabilitation nach Schlaganfall. Kohlhammer, Stuttgart

Pashkow P (1996) Outcomes in cardiopulmonary rehabilitation. Phys Ther 76:643–656

Peel C (1996) The cardiopulmonary System and movement dysfunction. Phys Ther 76:448–468

Sadowsky HS (1996) Cardiac transplant: a review. Phys Ther 76:498–515

Sayre, RS, Marcoux BC (1992) Exercise and autologous bone marrow transplants. Clin Manage Phys Ther 12(4):78–82

Simionato R, Stiller K, Butler D (1988) Neural tension signs in Guillain-Barré syndrome: two case reports. Aust J Phys Ther 34(4):257–259

Teasdale G, Jennett B (1974) Assessment of coma and impaired consciousness. Lancet 7:81–83

Umphred DA (ed) (1995) Neurological rehabilitation, 3rd edn. Mosby, St. Louis

Welch E, Anastasas M (1996) Critical care, critical choice. PT Magazine Phys Ther 3:75–77

Ziegler A (1996) Kommunikation mit Bewußtlosen. Vereinigung der Bobath-Therapeuten Deutschlands 30:7:2–19

11 Orthopedic and Sports Medicine

OBJECTIVES

By the end of this chapter the reader will be able to:
- Use the Swiss ball after *anterior cruciate ligament* (ACL) reconstruction and other lower extremity injuries/surgeries
- Treat patients with acute and chronic shoulder problems using the Swiss ball
- Apply treatment with the Swiss ball to patients with back instabilities and postural deficits
- Select exercises with the Swiss ball for patients with scoliosis
- Use the Swiss ball for proprioceptive and balance training with orthopedic patients

11.1 Introduction

Effective use of the Swiss ball with orthopedic patients requires the therapist to understand the underlying pathology. It is important that the therapist has a clear understanding of how the injury occurred, and what movements cause pain, including resting or working positions. The therapist can then evaluate these positions and make adaptations. Patients (especially those suffering back pain) who have less pain when moving (walking, skiing, exercising, etc.) and more pain when sitting or standing may benefit from Swiss ball exercises because *the ball is a dynamic tool.*

> The therapist must be aware of all precautions and contraindications with a particular orthopedic problem.

Precautions may vary considerably not only in regard to the particular joint but also the injury sustained and the surgery performed to repair it. Choosing which technique to use also depends on the physician who carried out the surgery, his point of view, and his experience. Therapists are frequently requested to follow a protocol suggested by the physician. Unfortunately many protocols are rather limited and do not incorporate the most recent knowledge about recovery from injuries and surgeries. Most protocols lack proprioceptive and skill training and frequently are boring and a poor motivator for the patient.

It is not surprising to find in reviewing cases of ACL reconstruction that *patients who do not follow a set protocol progress at a faster pace than those who do.* This finding has led to considerable changes in treatment protocols for ACL reconstruction (De Carlo et al. 1992; Shelbourne and Nitz 1990; Shelbourne et al. 1992). The new treatment approach is commonly known as accelerated rehabilitation after ACL reconstruction.

Recent studies emphasize impairment of proprioception after injuries or surgeries to the upper and lower extremities (Lephart et al. 1992, 1994; Corrigan et al. 1992; Smith and Brunolli 1989). Lephart et al. (1994) describe proprioception as a sensory afferent feedback mechanism which encompasses the sensation of joint motion (kinesthesia) and the joint position sense; disruption of the proprioception mechanism (of the shoulder joint) results in disruption of the normal neuromuscular reflex joint stabilization, which may contribute to excessive strain of the capsule and ligaments and the potential for continuing injury. Alvemalm et al. (1996) found a significant difference between kinesthesia of the shoulder joint measured in normal subjects and that in subjects with a history of frank anterior dislocation. Glencross and Thornton (1981) tested position sense after ankle injuries and found that normal functioning of the joint in skilled actions is likely to be inadequate as a result of the distortion of proprioceptive signals.

Janda (1996) also stresses the importance of restoration of proprioception after injuries. He states that injuries to joints typically occur at the end of a sport game when fatigue sets in, and recruitment of motor units is impacted. Increased proprioceptive input activates afferents to the central nervous system (CNS) and consequently improves efferent output (quality of movement) and may therefore prevent further injuries. It is interesting to find that bracing (with a sleeve type brace) improves proprioception (McNair et al. 1996). This may explain why many patients like wearing a sleeve-type support after injuries or even continue for a long time to ace-wrap a sprain. Neutral warmth may also decrease firing of pain fibers and bring some pain reduction while increasing joint stability.

Strength and/or endurance of muscles is affected by altered input from sensory neurons (Lee 1994). A mild effusion in knee joints can stimulate mechanoreceptors in the capsule, synovium, or ligaments, inhibiting the vastus medialis oblique muscle activity in normal, asymptomatic subjects. Janda (1996) supports this idea, observing that altered information from the periphery results in altered information from the CNS, even when the change is painless. Consequent changes in muscle tone/atrophy follow a predictable, not accidental, pattern of muscle imbalances.

> Caution: Therapists treating orthopedic patients should remember that limitations of ROM can be due to joint versus muscle/fascia versus CNS tone. The CNS can affect ROM, for example, through fear of what the therapist may do and through lack of information (e.g., the physician telling the patient, after looking at the radiography "there is nothing wrong with you" while the patient's muscles are hurting). Simply by talking to the patient the therapist may be able to dispell the patient's fear; accepting the patient's feeling of pain may increase his ROM.

Therapists should also remember that muscle strength in non-CNS problems is truly a problem of strength. Once the CNS becomes involved, an increase in strength does not help unless it is available to the CNS.

> Since the CNS does not recognize individual muscles, but only movement patterns, the chances for a carryover depend on functional movement patterns. The closer the therapist can come to selecting patterns which the CNS must run, the greater is the likelihood for carryover (Umphred 1997, personal communication).

Working with a patient in a pleasant environment in a room with a balanced temperature, and giving the patient quality time in an atmosphere of trust can all affect the CNS of the patient and thus contribute to increased function (Umphred 1995, and personal communication).

Janda (1996) suggests three additional steps to improve the CNS function:
- Improve afferent input (proprioception)
- Maintain good posture/equilibrium (activation of cerebellum, vestibular system and spinal pathways)
- Activate deep intrinsic muscles of the trunk through old phylogenetic movements such as reflex crawling and reflex turning (Vojta 1981) and pressure points, triggering reflex responses

The third of these points is especially important in patients with back pain since the deep intrinsic muscles of the back act as stabilizers and cannot be activated voluntarily (Janda 1996). Reactive muscle training with the Swiss ball may help activate the intrinsic back muscles since entire chains of muscles are involved in stabilizing and maintaining balance. When exercising the trunk muscles (for example, while lying prone over the ball) the therapist must observe the movement and give proper instructions to target the area which requires stabilization in order to prevent the movement from continuing or becoming an evasive movement. Active buttressing (see Sect. 5.8) and good conditios (Sect. 6.4) are especially useful when performing stabilization exercises for the back with or without the Swiss ball (Oehl 1996). Exercises such as The "Scale" and "Figurehead" require active buttressing.

All the above information confirms the importance of integrating the Swiss ball in treatments of orthopedic patients. The use of the Swiss ball is very functional because it allows the patient to do what he likes and to exercise at the same time. For example, if a patient enjoys watching TV, exercises which require sitting on the ball may have a functional carryover for sitting. The same activity can also be used to make the activity of watching TV a cognitive distraction in order to run procedural/automatic programs.

> Caution: If exercises of alternate leg movements at gait velocity are performed in supine position while watching TV, the patient must then stand up and walk to obtain a functional carryover. The Swiss ball can be used in the patient's bed or the living room so that he does not have to travel to a gymnastic establishment in order to exercise, but, as mentioned above, a functional activity should follow the exercises.

The Swiss ball can be used with orthopedic patients to:
- Perform a global assessment
- Increase ROM of the trunk and extremities
- Strengthen the trunk and extremities. It is a great tool for closed kinetic chain exercises
- Train proprioception
- Train muscle skill and balance
- Position the affected extremity
- Practice alignment
- Reduce the weight of a body segment or part thereof
- Achieve reactive muscle training
- Motivate the patient
- Perform manual therapy

Chapter 7 presents examples of how to use the Swiss ball to test and improve ROM, strength, balance, and alignment. Chapter 6 describes states of muscle activity and reactive training (actio-reactio principle), and Chapter 5 discusses the critical points of observation. Examples for manual therapy are provided in Sect. 8.5.

In the following section the example of ACL reconstruction and rehabilitation is used to explain the benefits of using the Swiss ball for exercises of the lower extremities. It is easy for the therapist to find applications of some of these exercises for patients with total hip or knee replacement (see also Fig. 7.3) if precautions are observed. Exercises can be designed for many lower extremity conditions. Recently a patient suffering from severe patellafemoral problems told me: "I did not like doing the exercises I was given by the therapist as homework, but since I've been using the Swiss ball it is fun, and I enjoy exercising and am improving."

11.2 After ACL Reconstruction

Stanish and Lai (1993) review ACL rehabilitation and provide a scientific basis for the rehabilitation program after reconstruction of a torn ACL. These authors note that pain is the primary concern during the initial phase (0–2 weeks postoperatively) of rehabilitation. The surgical trauma and pressure from the swelling stimulates sensory pain fibers. Other authors agree about the importance of addressing joint effusion in the early rehabilitation phase whether the reconstruction was performed from a patellar autograft or allograft (Shelbourne et al. 1992; Mangine and Noyes 1992). All the above authors agree with Wilk and Andrew (1992) that during the first 7–10 days the patient should obtain passive knee extension, be able to perform a visible quadriceps set (active contraction to mobilize the patella and to prevent infrapatellar scarring), and ambulate safely with crutches wearing a brace locked at 0° extension.

At least 90° knee flexion should be achieved during the first 2 weeks after surgery. Shelbourne et al. (1992) refer to *full knee extension as the ability to hyperextend the knee to the same degree as the normal knee.* They encourage the patient to limit walking during the first 2 weeks and to keep the leg elevated. The wound must be healed before the patient progresses to the next phase. The patient walks with a knee immobilizer until day 7 and is then fitted with a double-hinged knee brace (Shelbourne et al. 1992). None of the authors mention either proprioception and alignment exercises or the use of the Swiss ball in the early phase of recovery.

The benefit of the Swiss ball is seen in the following:
1. The patient is challenged to keep the leg aligned while moving it.
2. The patient is in control of the movement. Initially the unaffected leg can help move the ball, and the patient then progresses to performing the flexion/extension movement unassisted, in good alignment with the affected leg.
3. The patient receives feedback by observing his ability to move the leg in a straight line from flexion to extension.
4. The patient is motivated because moving the operated leg with reduced weight often decreases the pain.
5. Unlike the continuous passive motion machine, the Swiss ball can easily be moved from the bed to the living room or the den, wherever the patient wishes.
6. The tool is very cost effective.
7. The Swiss ball can be used immediately after surgery to elevate the leg.

11.2.1 1–3 Weeks After ACL Reconstruction

> *Figure 11.1a.* A 16-year-old female patient 7 days after ACL recon-
> struction to the right knee has her leg elevated on the Swiss ball
> while working on extending the knee passively. Dots are placed on
> knee and foot to create an awareness of alignment.

This position is beneficial because gravity assists both venous and lymphatic
return. Because the ball can be placed more proximally (Fig. 11.1b) or more
distally, the patient can adjust for comfort. If the ball is placed more distally,
the effect is passive knee extension similar to towel extension (De Carlo et al.
1992), with the advantage of having the leg elevated at the same time. The
patient can perform active ankle pumps with the legs elevated.

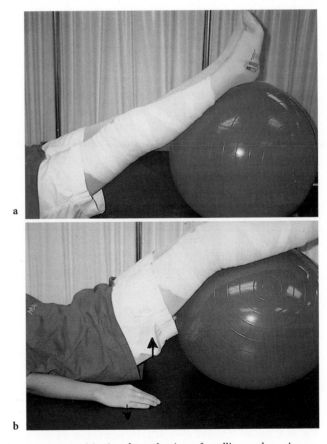

Fig. 11.1 a, b. A patient demonstrates positioning for reduction of swelling and passive extension 7 days after ACL reconstruction of the right leg.

Personally, I also instruct the patient how to activate the lymph system manually by using lymph drainage strokes on the inside of the thigh (Carrière 1988). Of course, ice can be placed on the knee, which is recommended by the above authors, and its benefit is confirmed by a recent study (Albrecht et al. 1996).

EXAMPLES

Figure 11.2. A 27-year-old patient 3 weeks after ACL reconstruction demonstrates how to work on passive knee extension while sitting on a chair/sofa (e.g., when watching TV at home). Alignment of the knee and foot are encouraged. Dots are placed on the knee and the second ray of the toe to give visual feedback. Early awareness of alignment is important to reduce patella-femoral problems after surgery.

Figure 11.3. The positions demonstrated in Figs. 11.1 and 11.2 are also the starting positions for active knee flexion. The Swiss ball reduces the weight of the affected leg, and the unaffected leg can act as a mover of the ball. Active flexion and extension of the knee are practiced in good alignment.

The therapist can give gentle resistance to the ball to increase the demand on the hamstring muscles. A continuous passive motion machine, on the other hand, is a passive device which does not correct alignment and does not necessarily do what it is supposed to do. Recently a colleague shared a story which emphasizes this point. She had seen a patient who was put in a passive motion machine machine set at 0°–30° after knee surgery (tibia plateau fracture). Many hours later it was discovered that by mistake the hinged knee brace was locked the entire time in extension while the passive motion machine machine was "flexing" the knee.

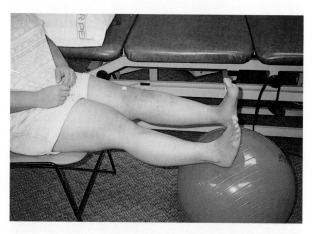

Fig. 11.2. Patient 3 weeks after ACL reconstruction on the left knee works on extension (and flexion) of knees and hips while sitting in a chair. The legs are supported by the Swiss ball.

The Swiss ball can be used to support the knees in flexion while activating the hip extensor muscles in a bridge activity. Strong hip extensor (and hip abductor) muscles are important for normal gait. When lifting the pelvis the hip abductor muscles must assist to maintain balance. The back extensor muscles must also stabilize.

EXAMPLES

Figure 11.1b. The same patient as in Fig. 11.1a demonstrates active hip extension in a bridge activity 7 days postoperatively.

As soon as the patient can sit, a Swiss ball can be used instead of a chair.

The benefit of using the Swiss ball instead of a chair is:
8. To challenge balance
9. To practice alignment while balancing on the ball
10. To increase awareness of symmetrical weight bearing
11. Proprioceptive training when bouncing gently
12. The ability to flex the knee from the proximal lever
13. To self-correct and receive instant feedback

An insecure patient may feel safer when sitting at first on a PhysioRoll because the base of support is greater, and the double ball cannot roll to the side. When a Swiss ball is chosen, it must be large enough to compensate for the available ROM of the knees and patient's proportions (Carrière and Felix 1993). At first it is important for the patient to sit at least 90°–90° hip and knee flexion, perhaps between chairs for his safety. A mirror placed in front of the patient enables him to correct the alignment.

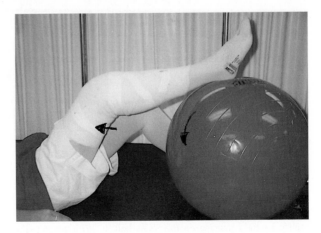

Fig. 11.3. Patient flexes her knee using the Swiss ball 7 days postoperatively.

EXAMPLES

Figure 11.4. Panel a. The patient demonstrates poor alignment 3 weeks post surgery. This malaligned position could explain the biomechanical stress causing patella-femoral pain. If the vastus medialis oblique muscle is weakened, the patella cannot track correctly, and if the leg is not properly aligned, joint congruency may also not be optimal. Note that with this closed kinetic chain activity the weight bearing of the lower extremities is not symmetrical.

Panel b. The patient has corrected the alignment and weight bearing on the operated (left) leg. In this position the patient can begin gentle bouncing (proprioceptive training) and pull the ball toward the heels to strengthen the hamstring muscles. The patient can push back with the unaffected leg or let the ball passively roll back in order to pull it forward again. The patient can learn to alternately take steps in good alignment.

The patient can also perform active quadriceps contractions with the knee resting on the Swiss ball in this phase of treatment. Shelbourne et al. (1992) state that this mobilizes the patella and places the patella tendon at length. Ab- and adduction of the hip joint with the weight of the legs supported on the ball can also be practiced.

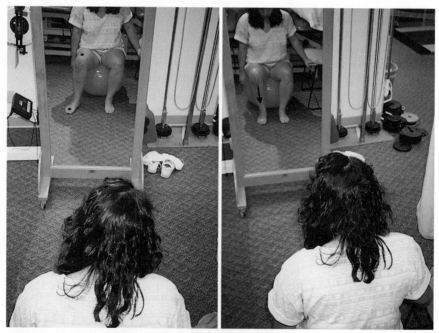

a   b

Fig. 11.4 a. Patient 3 weeks after ACL reconstruction sitting in poor alignment and nonsymmetrical weight bearing on the Swiss ball. **b.** With corrected alignment and weight bearing for proprioceptive training in closed kinetic chain.

11.2.2 3 Weeks After ACL Reconstruction

At the end of 2 weeks the patient should be able to extend the knee passively completely, perform a straight leg raise with a slight lag without difficulty, and have only minimal swelling (Shelbourne and Wilckens 1990). The second phase (2–5 weeks postoperatively) involves increasing flexion (to 120° or more by 5 weeks), developing a functional gait and resuming activities of daily living. Shelbourne et al. (1992) reformulated the phases, considering phase 1 to be preparation for surgery and phase 2 as the period up to 3 weeks post surgery, after which the third phase begins. At this time the patient should be able to walk without aids and without a limp (Shelbourne et al. 1992).

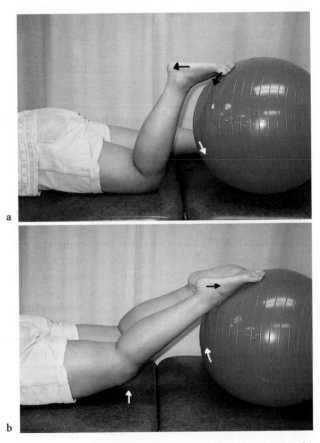

Fig. 11.5 a. Three weeks after ACL reconstruction the patient is actively strengthening the hamstring and dorsiflexor muscles. **b.** The quadriceps muscles are strengthened in prone in a bridge activity.

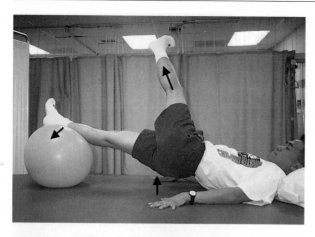

Fig. 11.8. A patient demonstrates the stabilizing variation of the "Pendulum" (reprinted from Carrière (1993) Swiss Ball exercises PT magazine. Phys. Ther. 9:92–100, with permission of the APTA)

11.2.3 More than 5 Weeks After ACL Reconstruction

The final phase of the rehabilitation process begins 5 weeks postoperatively, at which time the strength in the affected leg should be about 70% of that in the unaffected leg. At this time Shelbourne et al. (1992) introduce running, cariocas, rope jumping, and lateral shuffles. Wilk and Andrew (1992) begin straight leg raises in all planes 2–6 weeks postoperatively and begin walking without a brace when quadriceps strength is 60% of that in the other leg. O'Meara (1993) emphasizes weight training with the quadriceps, adductor, and hamstring muscles.

None of the above exercises train skill adequately. This was demonstrated by patients in a group ACL class, a few of whom who were already lifting weights and ambulating without a brace 6 or more weeks after surgery. They observed my patient doing Swiss ball exercises and tried themselves to perform the exercises – unsuccessfully, however, as they still lacked skill and coordination. It took time and effort for them to learn the exercises properly.

The patient in Figs. 11.1, 11.3, and 11.9–11.14 had three therapy sessions with me, 7 days, 3 weeks, and almost 6 weeks postoperatively. Each time she practiced the exercises at home in addition to coming to the ACL classes. The patient had good body awareness, obviously enjoyed exercising, and recovered well.

5–6 Weeks After ACL Reconstruction of the Right Knee

EXAMPLES

Figure 11.9. A 16-year-old patient demonstrates the "Cocktail Party" (Sect. 9.28). The right leg is in a closed chain and the left leg in an open kinetic chain. Both quadriceps muscles must work reactively to maintain balance. Good alignment and proprioception are trained when the patient changes the weight bearing from one leg to the other.

Figure 11.10. The "Scissors" (Sect. 9.19) requires straight leg raises in different planes, and both legs are in free-play function. In this end position the abductor muscles are trained in the upper leg while the adductor muscles are activated in the lower leg. The muscles work reactively.

Figure 11.11. The patient performs the exercise "Figurehead" (Sect. 9.18) and demonstrates good knee extension against gravity.

Figure 11.12. Practicing the "Sea Urchin" (Sect. 9.14), the patient achieves active knee and hip flexion by beginning the movement from the distal lever. The unaffected leg serves as main mover until the operated leg moves increasingly actively.

Figure 11.13. The exercise "Donkey Stretch Yourself" (Sect. 9.4) improves knee flexion from the proximal lever in a closed kinetic chain when changing from lying supine on the ball to leaning against the ball.

Figure 11.14. The exercise "Dolphin" (Sect. 9.29) demands stepping from side to side with the outer leg in good alignment and moving from a sitting position on the ball to a standing position on one leg. There is a constant change from open to closed kinetic chain with each step.

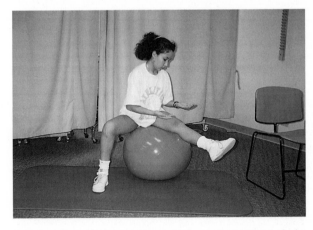

Fig. 11.9. Approximately 5–6 weeks after ACL reconstruction the patient mastered the "Cocktail Party".

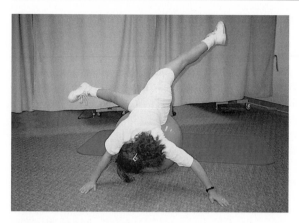

Fig. 11.10. The "Scissors" trains the lower extremities in all planes.

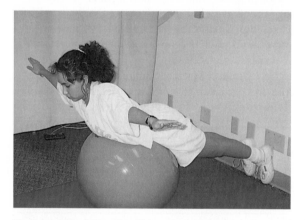

Fig. 11.11. The "Figurehead" is a closed kinetic chain exercise for the lower extremities.

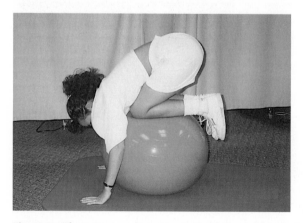

Fig. 11.12. The patient works on increasing knee and hip flexion with "Sea Urchin." The unaffected leg moves the ball until the involved leg can perform it.

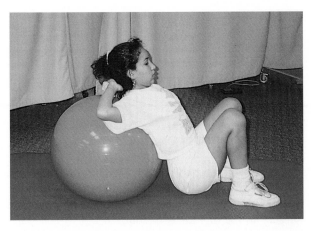

Fig. 11.13. The "Donkey Stretch Yourself" helps to improve knee flexion from the proximal lever.

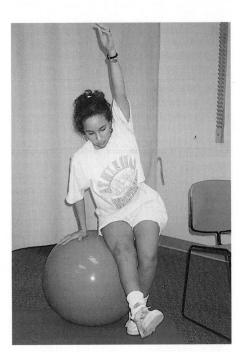

Fig. 11.14. The "Dolphin" trains weight shifting from one leg to the other changing from closed to open kinetic chain in good alignment.

All the above exercises (in addition to Figs. 7.24–7.26) can be incorporated into a treatment protocol if precautions are observed. The patient's safety should always be the therapist's concern, and there should be no increase of pain. There may be indications to perform manual therapy in the course of recovery. Examples are given in Figs. 8.14–8.16.

From their study of rehabilitation of the ACL in athletes, Silfverskiold et al. (1988) conclude that no rehabilitation should be used as a "cookbook recipe," and that rehabilitation should be fun. The ultimate goal is always the patient's well being and safe return to work and athletic activity. This is very important and should provide therapists with encouragement to try new exercises.

11.2.4 Adaptation of Exercises

Depending on the patient's age, general health, state of recovery, and the precautions required, many of the exercises included in this book can be adapted and given as a home exercise program following other injuries or surgery to the hip, knee, or foot.

> A home program should be one that patients can perform easily and safely in their own home without supervision (Sashika et al. 1996).

Studying a 6-week home program outcome for total hip arthroplasty 6–48 months after surgery, Sashika et al. (1996) concluded that the home program is effective at improving disabilities after total hip arthroplasty. The Swiss ball can be used safely with many patients. A Swiss ball can be used while resting in bed (e.g., performing "bridging" or flexion/extension exercises with the elevated legs), which is helpful in elderly patients. The Swiss ball can also be used while sitting in a chair.

> Proper alignment should be trained even before the patient is scheduled for surgery. The biomechanical integrity of a joint must be restored as soon as possible to avoid patellar tracking problems, increased swelling, pain and irritation of the knee, and unnecessary muscle imbalances.

The patient can learn to ambulate or rest the leg on the floor in good alignment (Fig. 11.15). The patient can practice sitting down and standing up in good alignment, his knees and feet marked with dots. He can also observe his alignment in a mirror placed in front of the stationary bicycle or any other equipment.

> Poor alignment is unfortunately a common problem but is often overlooked by physical therapists.

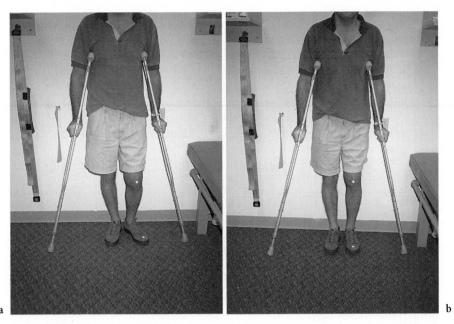

a   b

Fig. 11.15a,b. A patient demonstrates faulty and corrected alignment while standing supported by crutches.

11.3 After Shoulder Injuries and Surgeries

11.3.1 Introduction

The upper extremities are used predominantly in an open kinetic chain when walking and moving around. Perhaps for this reason open kinetic chain function pendulum exercises are popular both in Europe and the United States. Leaning forward while exercising, some patients suffer less pain when the weight of the arm is hanging and distracting the glenoid humeral shoulder joint. Pendulum exercises are often used to begin moving an injured shoulder (Kisner and Colby 1990). Many other exercises can be performed, and examples are provided by Kisner and Colby (1990), List (1996), and Bronner and Gregor (1992). Therapists may also draw ideas from Posner-Mayer's book (1995) on Swiss ball applications for orthopedic and sports medicine. Closed kinetic chain activity of the upper extremities is required when walking on the hands or pushing a heavy object.

The Swiss ball can be used in patients with acute and frozen shoulders for the following:
- To enable the patient to move the arm without having to lift it
- To increase the ROM of the shoulder by moving the proximal lever
- To decrease pain
- To let the patient rather than the therapist lift and move the painful arm
- To enable the patient to exercise at home while sitting on a sofa or standing in front of a table
- To achieve gentle compression (increased weight bearing on the hands) which usually does not increase the pain

When I first began using the Swiss ball several years ago for patients with injuries to the upper extremities, it was not evident to me why the patients liked the exercises and were very compliant. After years of experience some of the reasons have become apparent:

Swiss ball exercises may be important after injuries to the upper extremities because:
- The exercises are more functional, for they can easily be performed at home, and the patient can see the progress.
- Compression to the joint is important for stimulating the mechano-receptors to restore proprioception and neuromuscular joint stability, which is impaired after any injury or surgery (Smith and Brunolli 1989; Lephart 1994).
- Closed kinetic chain activity of the upper extremity requires coactivation of agonists and antagonists and may therefore protect the freshly injured joint better than open kinetic chain exercises.
- Muscle strength improves, which allows greater active ROM in open kinetic chain after the closed kinetic chain activity.

The example presented in the following section demonstrates these advantages.

11.3.2   Acute Nonsurgical Shoulder Injury

Figure 11.16. A 34-year-old man fell and injured his left shoulder. There was no fracture, and several days later the patient was referred to physical therapy for his shoulder pain and inability to move the arm.

Panel a. The patient was very apprehensive; initial measurements for active ROM were 20° forward flexion and 0° abduction of the left shoulder. After the patient lifted the left arm passively onto a small (45-cm) Swiss ball he was able to move it with the help of the other arm into forward flexion and horizontal ab- and adduction of the shoulder.

The patient was also instructed to keep the ball still and move the trunk away from the ball (shoulder flexion initiated from the proximal lever).

Panel b. The patient became confident and motivated and his mood changed when he realized that he could move his arm himself and the therapist was not causing him more pain. During the same first treatment session the patient was then instructed to perform closed kinetic chain exercises (support function) by doing minimal push-ups while lying on a 55-cm-diameter ball, a size which suited the length of the patient's arms.

Panel c. The patient's ROM improved to approximately 35° active forward flexion during approximately the first 10 minutes of practice.

Panel d. "Walking forward" on his hands, he increased the load on his shoulders, strengthened his arms, and challenged balance at the same time.

Panel e. He was then instructed to reduce the weight of the left arm which rested on the Swiss ball in order to "program" an open kinetic chain (free-play) activity of the injured arm. Using the Swiss ball in this way prevented the patient from fearing that he would not be able to lift the arm. The patient's hand position changed from thumb-up to thumb-down to activate different aspects of the upper arm muscles.

Panel f. The patient began wall slides with the ball.

Panels g, h. At the end of the first treatment the patient had gained approximately 50° of active movement (g) and more than 80° of passive movement with a minimal evasive movement visible at the left scapula (h). The patient took a 55-cm Swiss ball home to continue practicing as instructed.

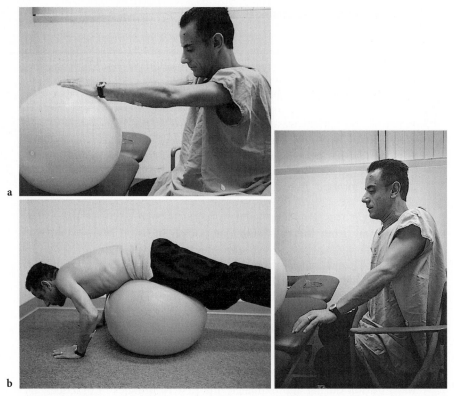

Fig. 11.16 a. Approximately 4 days after a fall onto the right shoulder a patient begins exercising with the Swiss ball (45 cm). **b.** During the same treatment session he is introduced to closed kinetic chain exercise (support function) lying prone over a 55-cm-diameter Swiss ball. **b.** After approximately 10 minutes the ROM had improved from 20° to about 35° forward flexion. **d.** Increasing the challenge by increasing the load on the left upper extremity and introducing balance of the trunk while exercising the shoulder. **e.** Beginning to strengthen the left upper extremity in an open kinetic chain by attempting to decrease the weight of the arm on the ball. **f.** Performing wall slides against gravity. **g.** Demonstrating increased active ROM at the end of the first treatment session. **h.** Demonstrating increased passive ROM, but still a slight evasive movement at the left scapula.

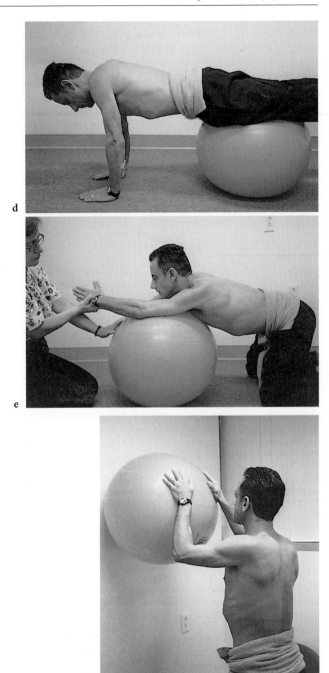

Fig. 11.16 d–f.

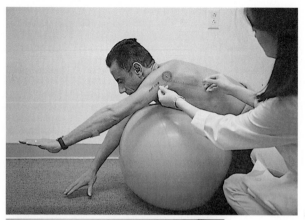

g

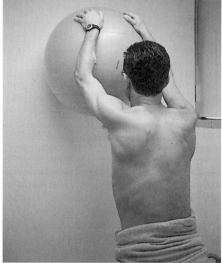

h

Fig. 11.16 g, h.

11.3.3 The "Frozen" Shoulder (Adhesive Capsulitis)

Patients often do not know the exact cause of their shoulder pain and immobility. Only sometimes can the patient remember a strain or injury to the shoulder preceding the onset of pain. The situation is depressing to the patient, and the limited use of the arm is very debilitating.

The patient may require joint and soft tissue mobilization as well as exercises to strengthen and stretch the arm to keep it from "freezing up" even further. It is important to carry all treatment out gently in order not to inflict further injury. The Swiss ball is a valuable tool for "frozen" shoulders. Patients enjoy using the ball and find it fun to exercise with. Several years ago when the Swiss ball was hardly known or used for shoulder treatments, a group of our patients was exercising using various Swiss balls. A patient who was waiting for treatment saw the group having fun and complained to the administration that we were "playing around" instead of exercising.

All the above exercises can be performed with patients who have various shoulder conditions, including the "frozen" shoulder. Some patients benefit from manual therapy. Figure 8.17 illustrates the use of the Swiss ball for manual therapy; further examples are provided in Chap. 8 for the patient as he progresses and can begin using assistive devices.

11.3.4 After Surgical Repair of the Shoulder

> Therapists should understand that the pathology of shoulder dysfunction usually differs in patients under 35 years from those over 35.

Young athletes often have injuries from overhead movements which may lead to instability, subluxation, and rotator cuff tears while older patients usually have shoulder disorders which result from the degenerative aging process (Jobe and Pink 1993).

After a rotator cuff injury or repair patients usually follow a protocol.

> It is very important in any rehabilitation program to avoid excessive anterior translation of the humeral head until dynamic joint stability is restored (Brewster and Moynes Schwab 1993).

Early pendulum exercises and passive ROM flexion and abduction are usually allowed, in addition to internal and external rotation of the arm with the elbow extended and at the side of the body. Active ROM begins 4–6 weeks after surgery (Kisner and Colby 1990; Brewster and Moynes Schwab 1993). Isometric exercises for internal/external rotation, abduction flexion, and extension are also commonly part of the program. Many clinics have their own protocols. To ensure proper healing the therapist must know which movements are contraindicated before applying Swiss ball exercises.

EXAMPLES

Figure 11.17. A patient 9 weeks after a surgical rotator cuff repair of the left shoulder. The goals: to increase ROM for forward flexion and abduction and to strengthen the shoulder muscles. The patient uses the PhysioRoll because he feels more secure with the increased base of support, the groove in the middle of the ball serves as a guide, and it rolls in only two instead of many directions.

Panel a. The patient moves the left arm, which was operated on 9 weeks earlier for a rotator cuff repair, on a PhysioRoll into abduction of the shoulder. In the end position the patient tries to decrease the weight of arm on the ball to strengthen the deltoid muscles. The pa-

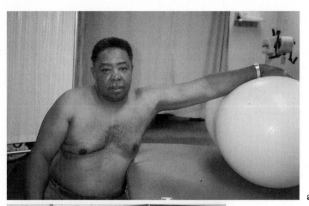

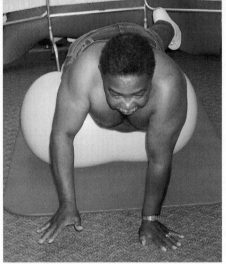

a

b

Fig. 11.17 a. Nine weeks after a rotator cuff repair the patient is using the Physio-Roll to increase the ROM for abduction of the shoulder. b. Strengthening his upper extremities, the left in a closed and the right in an open kinetic chain.

tient also exercised facing the PhysioRoll, placing one or both arms on top and moving the arms or the trunk to increase shoulder forward flexion.

Panel b. The patient is lying in prone position over the PhysioRoll, raising the left leg and the right arm to increase weight bearing on the left arm. The patient then lifts both legs while bearing weight alternately on the right and left arms and when "walking forward" on his hands, increasing the weight which is supported by the shoulder girdle. For "pushups" proper conditios ensure joint protection.

 To avoid excessive anterior translation of the humeral head the trunk should not be lower than the elbow level during the descent phase of a "pushup" (Brewster and Moynes Schwab 1993).

Bearing weight on his upper extremities, the patient could also keep his hands planted firmly on the floor and push the ball and trunk away while lowering the shoulders to increase the range of forward flexion. When the patient has mastered the exercises and is more confident, he can progress to performing the exercises on a Swiss ball, often during the first session (see also Fig. 12.1).

11.3.5 Additional Exercises for the Shoulder

Other exercises which can be performed as the shoulder heals and skill and strength training is emphasized in the program include: the "Goldfish" (Sect. 9.15), "Sea Urchin" (9.14), "Drunken Sea Urchin" (for horizontal ab- and adduction of the shoulder from the proximal lever), "Walking on Hands" (9.16), "Push Me–Pull Me" (9.17), "Scissors" (9.19), "Swing" (9.10), and "Salamander" (9.9). All of these exercises are in closed chain activity or support function. The "Figurehead" (9.18), "Scale" (9.2; variation with arm movements), and "Dolphin" (9.29) are exercises with open kinetic chain activity or play function. Before the patient is allowed to resume sports activities, the therapist can select from these exercises whichever she feels are safe for the patient to perform (see Chap. 9).

If precautions are observed, the Swiss ball can be used effectively not only with patients who require rotator cuff rehabilitation but also with patients following total shoulder arthroplasty. The therapist must be familiar with current treatment protocols (Brems 1994).

> All the patients whom I personally have treated after receiving a Neer prosthesis had sustained severe soft tissue injuries which presented greater problems than the prosthesis itself.

> The benefit of introducing the Swiss ball in the rehabilitation of the injured and repaired shoulder is that the trunk is supported by the PhysioRoll or the Swiss ball and, if performed correctly, there is no stress to the anterior aspect of the shoulder.

Proprioception can be addressed in the early stages of recovery as well as isometric exercises which may help to restore the neuromuscular joint stability.

> **The therapist must use her judgment when altering current treatment concepts. She must understand the purpose and the goal of the treatment and discuss the changes with the surgeon.**

11.4 Posture

11.4.1 Introduction

The restoration of a good shoulder/neck function includes the restoration of good posture. A stable, aligned trunk serves as a solid base for the shoulder girdle and neck. The shoulder girdle requires this solid base to avoid creating any stresses, imbalances, and altered movement pattern to the muscles surrounding the shoulder.

Few patients have pain of postural origin alone, but the postural component must be eliminated before an underlying mechanical cause can be identified (Grant and McKenzie 1994). Sahrman (1993) emphasizes the importance of looking at the musculoskeletal and nervous systems in addition to biomechancial factors.

> Only if the movement system is balanced can musculoskeletal pain be corrected.

Sahrman (1993) observes that altered length-tension properties of muscles is a base element fault of the musculoskeletal system, and that the interaction of various elements of the movement system is very important. Altered length tension properties of muscles are due to a base element fault of the musculoskeletal system. A nervous system fault is an alteration in the recruitment of synergies, while biomechanical (kinematic) faults result in a deviation of gravitation forces and patterns of muscle recruitment. White and Sahrman (1994) note than that, "Incorrect alignment and/or faulty force transmission through the musculoskeletal system leads to maladaptation of components of that system. Correction of kinetics at an early stage would contribute to the normal development of bones and joints."

Muscle imbalance in children usually begins in the upper part of the body (in adults in the lower part), perhaps because the child's large and heavy head is supported by comparatively weak neck muscles, and because the center of gravity of the child's head is located forward (Janda 1994). Janda (1986) also states that decreased activity and resulting weakness of some muscles may be due to altered movement patterns and changed motor regulation and motor performance. He considers impaired central nervous motor programming as one of the most important preconditions for development of chronic pain syndromes, and it is reflected by changes in the muscle tone of the entire body (Janda 1991).

> Poor postural alignment and muscle imbalances should be corrected as soon as they are recognized.

The exercises "Cowboy" (Sect. 9.1), "Scale" (9.2), and "Indian Fakir" (9.3) are important for training elements of a good upright posture because the aligned trunk is moved reactively in space.

11.4.2 Postural Deficits

The patient in Figs. 11.18–11.21 was a 6-year-old boy referred to physical therapy for his poor posture. In a standing position his head was in a forward position over his feet. The trunk leaned backward and rotated to the left, and the shoulders were protracted. The legs were hyperextended, with the right leg rotated externally and in poor alignment because the right lower leg was rotated more than the right thigh. The abdominal muscles were overstretched and weak, the pectoral muscles shortened, and the middle trapezius muscle was also very weak. The hip flexor muscles appeared tight; the hip extensor muscles were weak. The midthoracic spine lacked extension (Fig. 11.18a, first visit). Although the boy was cheerful and playful, he was somewhat shy and had poor body awareness and decreased balance and coordination.

The initial goal of the treatment was to familiarize the child with the Swiss ball in order to:
- Achieve good mobility of the spine (in all directions), and hip joints

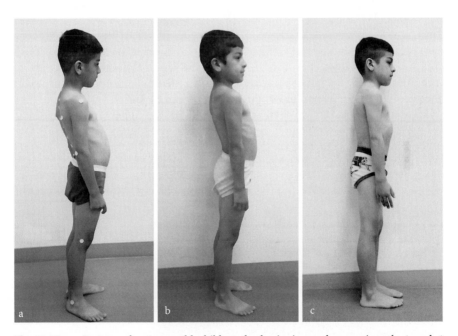

Fig. 11.18a–c. Posture of a 6-year-old child at the beginning and approximately 1 and 4 months after the initial treatment.

- Stretch the tight/shortened muscles playfully
- Strengthen the abdominal muscles
- Strengthen the back extensor and intrinsic muscles to stabilize the spine
- Strengthen especially the midtrapezius muscle in order to stretch the pectoral muscles
- Achieve symmetry of the trunk
- Increase body awareness and improve proprioception

The patient received a 45-cm Swiss ball for exercises at home but began many exercises on a small (red) PhysioRoll because of his poor balance and coordination. His mother was present during treatments (sometimes also his older brother) and was provided information about the findings and the goals. Photographs were taken at intervals of several weeks, and home exercises were modified during those sessions.

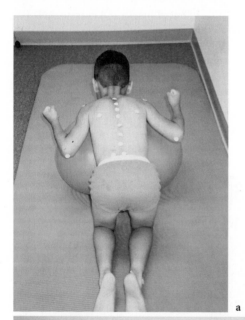

a

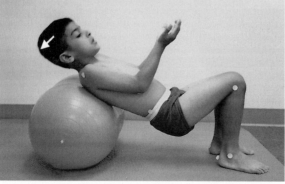

b

Fig. 11.19a,b. First session. a. Strengthening of the muscles of the midthoracic spine against gravity. b. The abdominal muscles and neck flexor muscles are strengthened. The child is supported by a PhysioRoll for increased support.

Figure 11.19. First session. Panel a. The patient strengthens the muscles of the midthoracic spine by supporting his trunk on a small PhysioRoll and lifting the flexed and externally rotated arms against gravity. (He also stretched his tight shoulders and mobilized the spine into extension while in prone position and resting his arms on a ball in front of him).

Panel b. Alignment of the head on the trunk is insufficient even when leaning against the PhysioRoll. The shoulders are protracted. The position of the arms helps to activate the abdominal muscles. The ventral neck muscles and the abdominal muscles must hold the weight of the head against gravity.

Figure 11.20. Panel a. First session. Lack of extension of the spine and tightness/weakness of the shoulder and trunk muscles is obvious when the patient attempts the exercise "Goldfish" (see Sect. 9.15). He can perform the exercise only on a small PhysioRoll.

Panel b. Approximately 4–5 months later (fourth treatment session). The patient can perform the exercise on a Swiss ball, he is able to lift the extended legs, back extension is improved, and forward flexion of the arm is increased.

Figure 11.21. Several weeks after the initial visit the boy returned for further instruction. His posture had improved (Fig. 11.18b, second session), and he had invented his own exercises. Panels a–f, second treatment session.

Panel a. He uses the ball actively to extend the spine, stretch his shoulders, and lift the head against gravity.

Panel b. He stretches his shoulders while resting the head in good alignment on the ball.

Panel c. With the trunk supported by the small PhysioRoll, he tries to lift his abducted and elevated arms against gravity with the hands behind the head.

Panel d. He is given a foam roll and attempts the "Sea Urchin" (Sect. 9.14) by pulling the legs under the trunk. This exercise strengthens especially the lower abdominal muscles and the shoulder girdle. Note that he chooses a wide base of support by keeping his knees apart (on his fourth visit he was able to keep his knees together while pulling the legs under the trunk).

Panel e. Lying on a foam roll and balancing the feet on a ball challenges alignment provides midline orientation and strengthens the trunk muscles.

Panel f. The patient (left) plays with his brother while strengthening his neck flexor and abdominal as well as the hamstring muscles.

Panel g. He learns to move the aligned and stabilized trunk forward while sitting on a Swiss ball (4th treatment session).

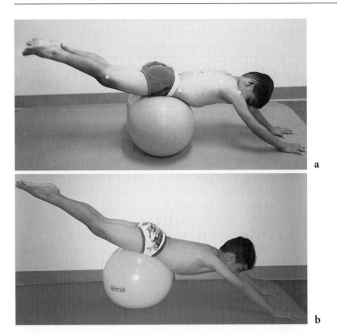

Fig. 11.20 a. First session: the patient has difficulty performing the "Goldfish." He exhibits shortness, tightness and weakness of the trunk muscles and hip flexor and shoulder forward flexion muscles. **b.** Four to five months later he has gained strength, mobility and increased balance. He can perform the exercise on a Swiss ball, and hip extension and forward flexion are improved.

Approximately 4–5 months after the initial visit the patient returned for another session and again his posture was improved (Fig. 11.18c, fourth treatment). The child was followed for several more visits to fine-tune the exercises to be performed at home. As the patient gained strength, the exercises were made more challenging, for example, by adding assistive devices such as Thera-Band and by decreasing the base of support.

Many of these exercises can be performed with adults who have postural deficits. Pain from exercise remains a contraindication.

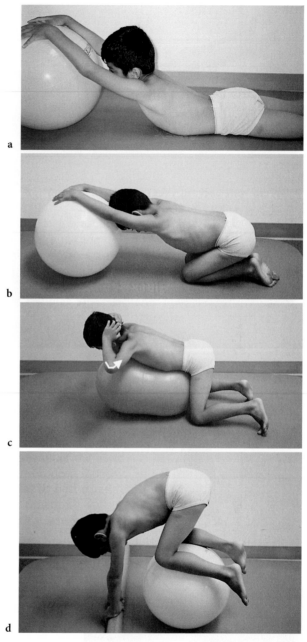

Fig. 11.21 a–f. Second session. **a–c.** the patient "invents" his own exercises to mobilize the spine into extension. **d.** The "Sea Urchin" is performed with a wide base of support. **e.** Strengthening the trunk muscles on a foam roll while balancing the feet on a ball. **f.** Playfully strengthening the abdominal, neck flexor, and hamstring muscles. **g.** Fourth treatment session. Learning to move the aligned and stabilized trunk forward while sitting on the Swiss ball.

EXAMPLES

Figure 11.25. Panel a. The patient performs the exercise "Walking on Hands" (see Sect. 9.16) to balance the two sides of the trunk while receiving tactile cues from the therapist. It is difficult for the patient to keep the ball rolling in a straight line and keep the legs on the Swiss ball.

Panel b. The patient pulls the legs under the trunk to reach the position of the "Sea Urchin" (see Sect. 9.14). The patient is then asked to perform the variation the "Drunken Sea Urchin" which requires moving the knees and the ball side to side, rotating the pelvis and lower trunk. The patient immediately finds out which side requires greater effort and feels challenged to make the sides feel equal.

Panel c. The therapist performs soft tissue mobilization of the posterior aspect of the trunk while the patient kneels in the end position of the "Sea Urchin." The patient can also breathe into the stretched posterior aspect of the trunk.

Panel d. The therapist gives the patient tactile cues to lower the shoulders, extend the back, and lift the legs (see the "Goldfish" Sect. 9.15). Strength, skill, and balance are required.

Panel e. The patient performs the "Swing" exercise (Sect. 9.10) loading and unloading the spine in a symmetrical position for proprioceptive training.

Panel f. An adaptation is made from a Klapp exercise to stretch the trunk. The right arm and head rest on a large Swiss ball and the right leg pulls in the opposite direction. The therapist can modify the direction of movement of the right arm and leg to achieve the best correction. The movement can then be compared with that of the other side. Sometimes it is advisable to practice only one side to correct the faulty movement and to achieve symmetry.

Panel g. Supine on the large (65-cm) Swiss ball the patient strengthens his abdominal muscles, especially the oblique ones on the left side. The therapist can give resistance and a tactile stimulus to improve muscle function.

There are many more exercises the patient can learn in several sessions, for example, the "Cowboy" (Sect. 9.1), "Scale" (9.2), "Indian Fakir" (9.3) "Figurehead" (9.18), and "Scissors" (9.19). Thera-Band can be used for exercises as described in Sect. 8.3 when the patient masters the exercises without weights or resistance.

Fig. 11.25 a. The exercise "Walking on hands" challenges balance of the trunk muscles. **b.** The patient is pulling the legs under the trunk training the abdominal muscles. **c.** Soft tissue mobilization can be carried out in the end position of the "Sea Urchin." **d.** Tactile cues help the patient to lower the shoulders and extend the back and legs. **e.** The "Swing" is good proprioceptive training for the spine. **f.** The patient stretches the trunk with an adapted Klapp exercise. **g.** Supine on the Swiss ball, the patient can train his abdominal muscles against gravity.

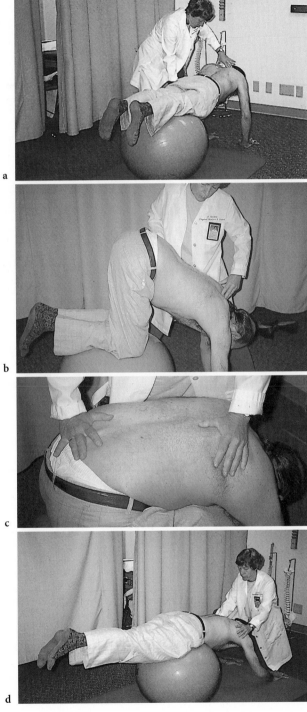

a

b

c

d

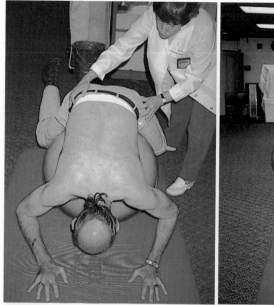
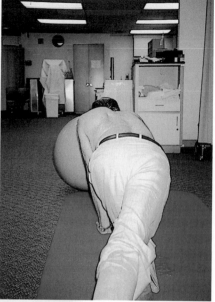

e

f

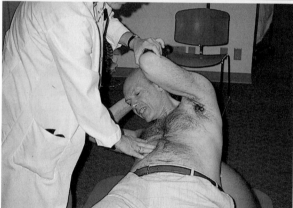

g

Abb. 11.25 e–g

Figure 11.26. Another adult patient with a severe scoliosis which compromises her breathing.
Panel a. The deformity of the spine is very obvious in sitting.
Panel b. A 55-cm Swiss ball is used to elongate the left side of the trunk. The patient pushes the ball forward with her left hand and slightly to the right side to achieve greater symmetry and to be able to increase ventilation of the left lower lobe of the lung.

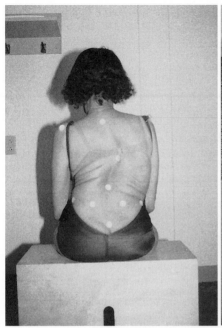

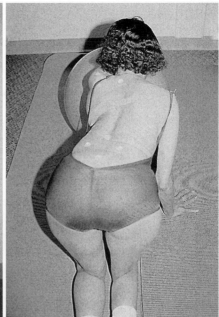

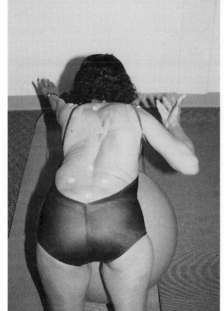

Fig. 11.26 a. Sitting posture of a adult patient with a severe scoliosis. **b.** The patient stretches her left side using the Swiss ball while supporting herself with the right arm. **c.** She supports her trunk on the ball to elongate the left side and strengthen the upper trunk. (From Carrière B (1996) Therapeutic exercise and self correction programs. In: Flynn TW (1996) The thoracic spine and rib cage. Butterworth-Heinemann, Boston, with kind permission from the publisher).

Panel c. The patient's trunk is supported by the Swiss ball and right arm supinated, flexed in the elbow, and externally rotated in the shoulder joint. The left arm is extended and the left side of the trunk elongated.

Figure 11.27. Panel a. An 18-year-old patient who suffered from cerebral palsy and severe scoliosis.

Panel b. The therapist uses a Swiss ball for herself, extending and elongating the trunk of the sitting patient.

Panel c. The patient is supported, and sits comfortably. The therapist can work on trunk and head control as well as on breathing exercises (view from the side).

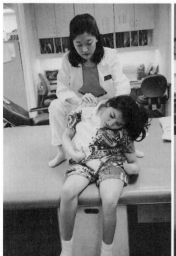

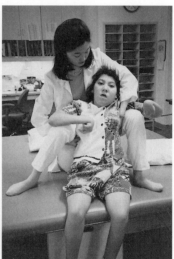

a

b

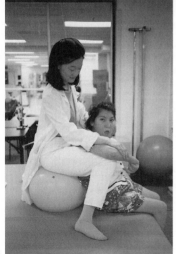

c

Fig. 11.27a–c. An 18-year-old patient with cerebral palsy and severe scoliosis. **a.** Sitting posture. **b.** The therapist is positioned on the Swiss ball to extend the trunk of the patient and elongate the left side of the trunk (view from the front). **c.** The patient is sitting comfortably, and the therapist can work on head and trunk control (view from the side).

There are many other Swiss ball exercises which can be incorporated into the treatment of a patient with a scoliosis. Many therapists choose exercises from different schools of thought to individualize the exercises to the patient's needs and abilities.

How complex and interwoven orthopedic, neurological, and gynecological problems can be illustrated by the following case study:

EXAMPLES

A previously healthy 9-year-old girl came for physical therapy with the following history (she was not referred for her incontinence problem). At the age of 5 years (1993) the girl had fallen from monkey bars in a playground. Her gait and posture slowly deteriorated, and the following year the family consulted an orthopedic physician. Magnetic resonance imaging showed a slipped disk and spondylolisthesis at L4-L5-S1. Because her symptoms worsened, a spinal fusion was performed in 1995. The patient had neither bladder nor bowel incontinence. A second operation was performed on her back in August 1996 because the initial surgery had been unsuccessful, and the patient's gait and posture had continued to deteriorate. After the second surgery the patient suffered a cauda equina syndrome. Four months later, when she was evaluated for physical therapy, the patient showed a loss of sensation in the peritoneal area and S2 and S3 distribution. She required in- and out-catheterization four times a day to drain her bladder. According to her mother there was no volitional contraction of the anal sphicter and no control of the bowel. The patient was able to walk, but her gait was similar to that of a patient with muscular dystrophy. The patient had grossly 2+/5 strength in her knee extensors, 3/5 in her hip flexors, hip flexors, hip extensors, and 3+/5 in her hip abductors. Her dorsi-/plantar flexors were within the normal range; the knee flexors, especially the hamstring muscles and the adductor muscles of the hips showed almost normal (4+/5) strength. The patient balanced her body on her shortened hamstring muscles, protracting her shoulders because of her inability to adjust her posture in the lumbar/hip region. She also had pain in the low back.

The patient and her family were extremely motivated and willing to come two or three times a week to physical therapy. The patient brought a diary to therapy and used it to note new exercises and to keep record of the exercises that she performed at home. She also kept a record of her catheterization, which she learned to carry out herself after several months of therapy. From the beginning the emphasis was placed on training not only her weakened muscles, especially those of the pelvic girdle and the legs, but also to address the problem of bladder and bowel incontinence.

After consulting with the parents the patient was given pictures of the pelvic floor. To enable her to visualize the muscles a skeleton was used to describe their position and function. She was instructed in the exercises as described in Chap. 14, and others were developed together with the patient for strengthening the pelvic floor muscles and to create a sensory awareness of the pelvic floor. Including the pelvic floor in her strengthening exercises and combining them with breathing exercises proved helpful. Conscious relaxation of the pelvic floor was also practiced. The patient was allowed to give the exercises her own personalized names to help her create a functional visual image. "Lean Forward and Roll" became "Short Belly–Long Belly" (Fig. 11.28). The patient renamed a pelvic floor exercise in supine position the "Pelvic Sit-Up," and another pelvic floor exercise developed from the exercise "Duck" was given the name "Scary Cat." The patient also practiced "Right Stop–Left Stop" (Fig. 11.29). The "Easter Bunny" was adapted to serve as a strengthening exercise for extremities and the pelvic floor (Fig. 11.30). "Kick and Kick" was adapted to strength her weak quadriceps muscles while strengthening the pelvic floor (Fig. 11.31).

The first noticeable improvement after approximately 4 weeks of treatment was control of the bowel, although the patient still required suppositories. At that time there was very little voluntary voiding; residuals remained high. After approximately 3 months of physical therapy the patient was beginning to void more frequently spontaneously after feeling fullness of her bladder; the residuals were more frequently lower than the volitional output. Her mother reported a mild contraction of the anal sphincter muscle when applying suppositories. Voiding was improved, especially after therapy. Wetness or dampness of pads was reduced to once in 3–4 days. All muscles previously tested had gained strength, the patient's posture and gait improved, as did the length of the hamstring muscles. She no longer relied on them to support her. The patient's general mobility had improved, and she no longer complained of back pain. She returned to school and continued physical therapy for further treatment of the pelvic floor and strengthening of the muscles of her trunk and the extremities.

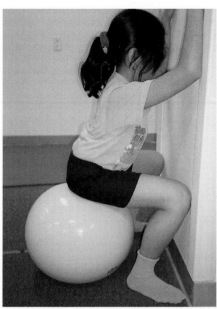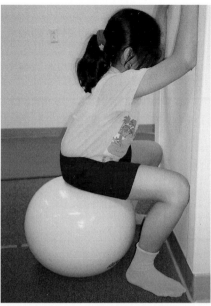

a   b

Fig. 11.28 a, b. "Long Belly–Short Belly" (see "Roll On," Chap. 14). **a.** "Long Belly." Inhalation and extension of the lumbar spine are combined with relaxation of the pelvic floor muscles. **b.** "Short Belly." Exhalation and flexion of the lumbar spine are combined with pelvic floor muscle contraction. Thorax and knees are spatially fixed points. The ischial tuberosities initiate the movement. The ball moves in a sagittal plane.

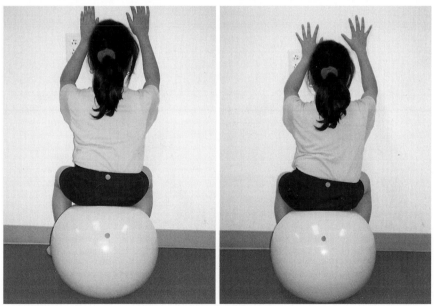

a   b

Fig. 11.29 a, b. The patient uses the same starting position as in Fig. 1a to move the ball in a frontal plane: from the center to the left side. Again the movement is initiated by the ischial tuberosities. (See "Right Top–Left Stop," Chap. 14).

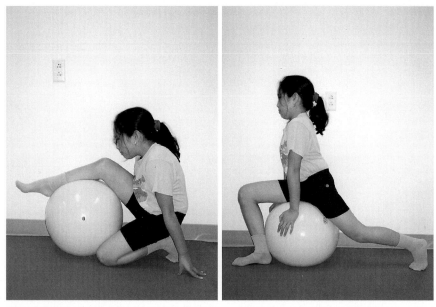

a   b

Fig. 11.30 a, b. The exercise "Easter Bunny" (Sect. 9.26) serves to move the ball in a sagittal plane, providing eccentric-concentric activity of the quadriceps (in the end position is a bridge activity). The patient also activates the pelvic floor muscles by pulling the ball with the ischial tuberosities toward the spatially fixed forward knee.

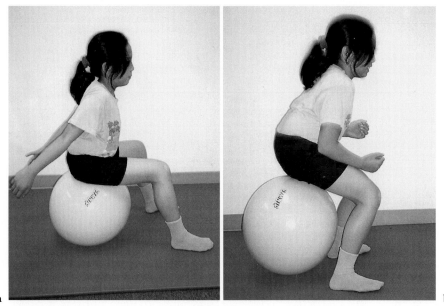

a   b

Fig. 11.31 a, b. The patient practices an adapted version of the exercise "Kick and Kick" (see Chap. 14) to strengthen the quadriceps muscles, mobilize the lumbar spine in flexion/extension, and train the fast-twitch fibers of the pelvic floor.

References

Albrecht S, Köhler V, Hardt F, Rossignol C, Le Blond R, Schlüter S (1996) Effiziens der kontinuierlichen Kryotherapie in der Frührehabiliation nach elektivem, endoprothetischen Hüftgelenkersatz. Krankengymnastik 48(8):1194–1202

Alvemalm A, Furness A, Wellington L (1996) Measurement of shoulder joint kinaesthesia. Manuelle Ther 1:140–145

Becker E (1987) Skoliosen-und Diskopathienbehandlung, 10th edn. Fischer, Stuttgart

Bold RM, Grossmann A (1989) Stemmführung nach R. Brunkow, 5th edn. Enke, Stuttgart

Brems, JJ (1994) Rehabilitation following total shoulder arthroplasty. Clin Ortho Relat Res 307:70–85

Brewster C, Moynes Schwab DR (1993) Rehabilitation of the shoulder following rotator cuff injury or surgery. J Orthop Sports Phys Ther 18(2):422–426

Bronner O, Gregor E (1992) Die Schulter und ihre funktionelle Behandlung, 2nd edn. Pfaum, München

Butler DS (1991) Mobilisation of the nervous system. Churchill Livingston, New York

Carrière B (1988) Edema: its development and treatment using lymph drainage massage. Clin Manage Phys Ther 8(5):19–21

Carrière Carrière B (1996) Therapeutic exercise and self correction programs. In: Flynn TW (1996) The thoracic spine and rib cage. Butterworth-Heinemann, Boston

Corrigan JP, Cashman WF, Brady MP (1992) Proprioception in the cruciate deficient knee. J Bone Joint Surg Br 74:247–250

De Carlo MS, Shelbourne KD, McCarroll JR, Retting AC (1992) Traditional versus accelerated rehabilitation following ACL reconstruction: a one year follow up. J Orthop Sports Phys Ther 15(6):256–364

Dreyer SJ, Dreyfuss PH (1996) Low back pain and the zygapophysial (facet) joints. Arch Phys Med Rehabil (77):290–300

Glencross D, Thornton E (1981) Position sense following joint injury. J Sport Med 21:23–27

Grant RN, McKenzie (1994) Mechanical diagnosis and therapy for the cervical and thoracic spine. In: Grant RN (ed) Physical therapy of the cervical and thoracic spine, 2nd edn. Churchill Livingstone, New York, pp 359–377

Hamilton C (1997) Segmentale Stabilisation der LWS. Krankengymnastik 49(4):614–622

Hamilton C, Richardson C (1997) Neue Perspektiven zu Wirbelsäuleninstabilitäten und lumbarem Kreuzschmerz: Funktion und Dysfunktion der tiefen Rückenmuskeln. I. Manuelle Ther 1:17–24

Hanke P (1991) Unterrichtsskript Krankengymnastische Behandlung auf entwicklungskinesiologischer Grundlage (unpublished)

Hardt I (1994) Behandlungsprinzipien und Wirkungsmechanismen der Skoliosebehandlung nach Vojta. In: Weiss HR (ed) Wirbelsäulendeformitäten. Fischer, Stuttgart, pp 41–45

Hennes A (1994) Behandlungsprinzipien und Wirkungsmechanismen der dreidimensionalen Skoliosebehandlung nach Schroth. In: Weiss HR (ed) Wirbelsäulendeformitäten. Fischer, Stuttgart, pp 67–72

Janda V (1986) Muscle weakness and inhibition (pseudoparesis) in back pain syndromes. In: Grieve GP (ed) Modern manual therapy of the vertebral column. Churchill Livingstone, New York, pp 197–201

Janda V (1991) Muscle spasm – a proposed procedure for differential diagnosis. J Manual Med 6:136–139

Janda V (1994) Muscles and motor control in cervicogenic disorders: assessment and management, 2nd edn. In: Grant R (ed) Physical therapy of the cervical and thoracic spine. Churchill Livingstone, New York, pp 195–215

Janda V (1996) Assessment of movement patterns in musculoskeletal disorders. Presented at the Workshop "Key Links to Musculoskeletal Dysfunction" at Kaiser Permanente Hospital, Los Angeles, 16–17 June, 13–14 August

Jobe FW, Pink M (1993) Classification and treatment of shoulder dysfunction in the overhead athlete. J Orthop Sports Phys Ther 18(2):427–432, 263–271

Kisner C, Colby LA (1990) Therapeutic exercises. Davis, Philadelphia

Klapp B (1990) Das Klappsche Kriechverfahren, 12th edn. Thieme, Stuttgart

Lee HWM (1994) Progressive muscle synergy and synchronization in movement patterns: an approach to the treatment of dynamic lumbar instability. J Manual Manipulative Ther 2(4):133–142

Lehnert-Schroth C (1975) Die Behandlung der Skoliose nach dem System Schroth. Krankengymnastik 9:322–327

Lehnert-Schroth C (1991) Dreidimensionale Skoliosebehandlung, 4th edn. Fischer, Stuttgart

Lehnert-Schroth C (1992) Introduction to the three-dimensional scoliosis treatment according to Schroth. Physiotherapy 78(11):810–815

Lephart SM, Kocher MS, Fu FH, Borsa PA, Harner CD (1992) Proprioception following ACL reconstruction. J Sports Rehab 1:188–96

Lephart SM, Warner JJP, Borsa PA, Fu FH (1994) Proprioception of the shoulder joint in healthy, unstable, and surgically repaired shoulders. J Shoulder Elbow Surg (3):371–80

List M (1996) Krankengymnastische Behandlung in der Traumatologie, 3rd edn. Springer, Berlin Heidelberg New York

Mangine RE, Noyes FR (1992) Rehabilitation of the allograft reconstruction. J Orthop Sports Phys Ther 15(6):294–302

McNair PJ, Stanley SN, Strauss GR (1996) Knee bracing: effects on proprioception. Arch Phys Med Rehabil 77(3):287–289

O'Meara PM (1993) Rehabilitation following reconstruction of the anterior cruciate ligament. Orthopedics 16(3):301–306

Ociepka R (1994) Skoliose-Korrekturgurt – ein neues Hilfsmittel zur Kräftigung der Muskeln der konvexen Seite der Verkrümmung. Krankengymnastik 46(7):925–928

Oehl M (1996) Die Bedeutung der aktiven Widerlagerung zur Stabilisation der Wirbelsäule. Krankengymnastik 48(5):694–701

Ozarcuk L (1994) Grundlagen der Skoliosebehandlung mit der propriozeptiven neuromuskulären Fazilitation in Weiss HR (ed) Wirbelsäulendeformitäten. Fischer, Stuttgart, pp 11–30

Posner-Mayer J (1995) Swiss ball applications for orthopedic and sports medicine. Ball Dynamics International, Denver

Sahrman SA (1993) Movement as a cause for musculoskeletal pain. In: Singer KP (ed) Integrating approaches. Proceedings of the Eighth Biennial Conference of the Manipulative Physical Therapists Association of Australia, 23–27 November, pp 69–74

Sashika H, Matsuba Y, Watanabe Y (1996) Home program of physical therapy: effect on disabilities of patients with total hip arthroplasty. Arch Phys Med Rehabil 77(3):273–277

Schneider G (1994) Behandlungsergebnisse der Skoliosebehandlung nach PNF in Weiss HR (ed) Wirbelsäulendeformitäten. Fischer, Stuttgart, pp 31–40

Shelbourne KD, Klootwyk TE, De Carlo MS (1992) Update on accelerated rehabilitation after anterior cruciate ligament reconstruction. J Orthop Sports Phys Ther 15(6):303–308

Shelbourne KD, Nitz P (1990) Accelerated rehabilitation after anterior cruciate ligament reconstruction. Am J Sports Med 18(3):292–299

Shelbourne KD, Wilckens JH (1990) Current concepts in anterior cruciate ligament rehabilitation. Orthopaedic review XIX (11):957–964

Silfverskiold JP, Steadman JR, Higgins RW, Hagerman T, Atkins JA (1988) Rehabilitation of the anterior cruciate ligament in the athlete. Sports Med 6:308–319

Smith RL, Brunolli J (1989) Shoulder kinesthesia after anterior glenohumeral joint dislocation. Phys Ther 69:106–112

Solomonow M, Baratta R, Zhou BH, Shoji EH, Bose W, Beck C, D'Ambrosia R (1987) The synergistic action of the anterior cruciate ligament and thigh muscles in maintaining joint stability. Am J Sports Med 15(3):207–213

Stanish WD, Lai A (1993) New concepts of rehabilitation following anterior cruciate reconstruction. Clin Sports Med 12(1):25–58

Umphred DA (1995) Limbic complex. In: Neurological rehabilitation, 3rd edn. Mosby, St. Louis, pp 92–117

Vojta V (1981) 3rd edn. Die zerebrale Bewegungsstörungen im Säuglingsalter. Enke, Stuttgart 114–146

Vojta V, Peters A (1992) Das Vojta-Prinzip. Springer, Berlin Heidelberg New York

Weiss HR (1991) Elektromyographische Untersuchungen zur skoliosespezifischen Haltungsschulung. Krankengymnastik 43(4):361–369

Weiss HR (1992) The progression of idiopathic scoliosis under the influence of a physiotherapy rehabilitation programme. Physiotherapy 78(11):815–821

Weiss HR (1994a) Der Verlauf unbehandelter idiopathischer Skoliosen, eine Literaturübersicht. In: Weiss HR (ed) Wirbelsäulendeformitäten. Fischer, Stuttgart, pp 1–9

Weiss HR (1994b) Behandlungsergebnisse der dreidimensionalen Skoliosebehandlung nach Schroth in der stationären Rehabilitation. In: Weiss HR (ed) Wirbelsäulendeformitäten. Fischer, Stuttgart, pp 73–80

White SG, Sahrman SA (1994) A movement balance approach to management of musculoskeletal pain, 2nd edn. In: Grant R (ed) Physical therapy of the cervical and thoracic spine. Churchill Livingstone, New York, pp 339–357

Wilk KE, Andrew JR (1992) Current concepts in the treatment of anterior cruciate disruption. J Orthop Sports Phys Ther 15 (6):279–293

Yack JH, Collins CE, Whieldon TJ (1993) Comparison of closed and open kinetic chain exercise in the ACL deficient knee. Am J Sports Med 21(1):49–53

12 Medical/Surgical Outpatient Care

OBJECTIVES

By the end of this chapter the reader will be able to:
- Use the Swiss ball with patients after mastectomy/lumpectomy
- Treat patients with postural deficits after surgeries
- Use the Swiss ball with patients who suffer from osteoporosis
- Select exercises for patients with ankylosing spondylitis

12.1 Surgical Patients

12.1.1 Introduction

A traumatic event such as an unexpected surgery or accident may cause emotional stress, pain, and a distorted self-image. Resulting physical limitations may prevent the patient from returning to work, earning a living, pursuing hobbies, and performing activities of daily living for an extended period of time. For example, after cancer resulting in a modified or radical mastectomy or lumpectomy, additional treatments such as chemotherapy or radiation may prolong the healing process; however, the patient may fear complications such as edema or recurrence of the cancer. Previously independent patients may become dependent on other persons to take them to therapy and help them at home, at least temporarily.

Patients, especially after major surgery (e.g., abdominal surgery), may lose considerable weight and feel stiff, weak, and tight around the chest. They experience difficulty in expanding the thorax. Patients can have sensory deficits, decreased kinesthetic awareness, pain, swelling, and decreased strength and endurance. Poor posture may be due either to the patient's emotional state or to tightness from surgical scars after injuries/repairs to the chest and trunk, or both.

Therapists treating these patients should have sympathy with the patient and a profound knowledge of the healing process and treatments of the structures involved.

The therapist must be sensitive to the patient's fears and be a good listener and observer. Some patients may try to hide their pain and fears while others are overly anxious to get well and need to be slowed down to prevent damage to the healing tissue.

12.1.2 Evaluation

The evaluation of postsurgical patients should include the following:
- Inspection of the scar and surrounding tissue for the integrity of the skin
- Inspection of skin temperature and possible swelling/edema
- Checking for sensory and proprioceptive/kinesthetic deficits
- Measurement of ROM
- Evaluation of soft tissue, neural tissue tension
- Evaluation of strength and endurance
- Evaluation of posture
- Determination of which functional movements can or cannot be performed

The therapist must know the patient's additional medical problems, his pain, which medications he is taking, and, in order to motivate him, his hobbies. This information helps the therapist to design exercises which are goal oriented and do not increase the pain.

> Patient and therapist must strive for a *common* functional goal which helps the patient to resume activities of daily living and to regain his independence.

Common goals also lead to compliance and the patient's active participation in the entire program.

Numerous treatment approaches described in previous chapters of this volume can be used to help these patients. Information on the patient's potential underlying problems after an injury or medical problem is presented by Flynn (1996), Cyriax (1982), List (1996), Travell and Simon (1983, 1992), and Umphred (1995). See also Chap. 10 for further references.

12.1.3 Treatment Approach

Treatment Goals

- Restore posture and alignment
- Increase joint, soft tissue and neural tissue mobility
- Increase strength and coordination
- Restore proprioception
- Achieve independence in a home exercise program
- Ability to resume activities of daily living and hobbies

Treatment Plan

The treatment plan is based upon evaluation, interpretation of evaluation results, and multiple system interactions:
- Strengthening exercises of trunk and extremities
- Mobilization of joints and soft tissue and neural structures
- Balance and coordination exercises combined with strengthening exercises
- Proprioceptive training
- Teach home exercise program

Precautions

- Allow wounds and scars to heal properly without pulling or tearing of the tissue.
- Check for lines or drains that the patient may still have months after the surgery.
- Note that radiated tissue loses its normal texture and can tear easily. Be gentle.
- After major surgery or injury the patient may be more labile and intolerant of vigorous treatments such as bouncing and quick change of position. It may be necessary to monitor blood pressure, heart rate, and respiration.
- Do not cause pain. Consider the patient's emotional state.
- Allow for an increased base of support when a patient is learning new exercises.
- Provide a safe environment.

Contraindication

 Never use heating pads or other heating devices with a patient whose lymph nodes have been removed because this can lead to lymphedema. Even taking hot baths or showers can be dangerous and trigger lymphedema (Carrière 1988). For example, do not put a hotpack on the patient's shoulder while performing stretching exercises with the Swiss ball if axillary lymph nodes have been removed.

12.1.4 Treatment Examples

The following treatment examples describe one patient after a mastectomy and another who underwent total abdominal surgery following a motor vehicle accident. In both cases the patient (or family) requested physical therapy when the extent of movement limitations and postural deficits was discovered.

Treatment examples for patients with adhesive capsulitis are presented in Chapter 11 because their treatment is usually prescribed by orthopedic physicians. All exercises described for shoulder patients in Chapter 11 can be performed with patients after a mastectomy, but the therapist may have to progress the patient more slowly because of the surgery. Although the surgical approach has changed in recent years and is now less aggressive (the pectorales muscle now is usually left intact), it can still be extensive in the case of a radical mastectomy.

Therapists should pay special attention to testing the serratus anterior muscle.

> Some patients suffer temporary (or permanent) *serratus anterior palsy after axillary node dissection* due to trauma or injury to the long thoracic nerve during surgery.

The palsy is often reversible (Duncan et al. 1983) and is more frequent in patients with radical modified mastectomy than in those with quadrantectomy (Gutman et al. 1990).

After Mastectomy

Two and a half months after a mastectomy (right side) the 50-year-old patient came for physical therapy because of a developing edema in her right arm. Although the patient followed a home program after surgery (written instructions given by nurses), in addition to the beginning edema, the mobility of her right shoulder had decreased.

The patient was treated primarily for her lymphedema but was also instructed in exercises with the Swiss ball to increase strength and mobility of her shoulder. Initially she complained of tightness of the right shoulder. ROM was limited to approximately 130° forward flexion and 70° for external rotation, with grossly fair muscle strength. Because of the patient's medium size she was provided with a 55-cm-diameter Swiss ball and exercises as described in Chapter 11 (Figs. 11.16, 11.17) and Chapter 2 (Fig. 2.11). Four weeks after the initial evaluation (3.5 months after her surgery) she demonstrated good functional movements and strength and was able to resume her activities of daily living but could not yet return to work as a surgical nurse because of continuing chemotherapy treatments.

EXAMPLES

Figure 12.1. Panel a. The patient moves her arms from the distal lever (see also Sect. 5.7), with the weight of the arm resting on the Swiss ball.

Panels b–d. She demonstrates movements from the proximal and distal lever and from the pivot point (the shoulder). By positioning the arm palm up or down the patient adds rotation to the movement (b,

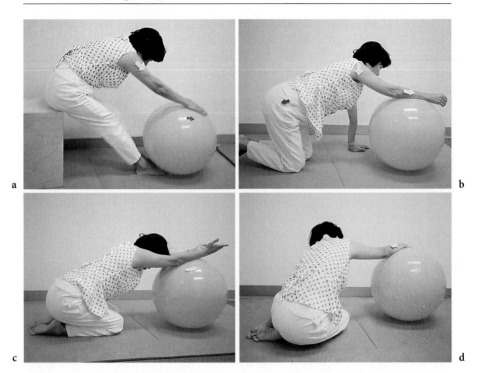

Fig. 12.1 a. The patient moves her arms from the distal lever. **b–d.** She demonstrates movements from the proximal and distal levers and as from the pivot point, the shoulder. **e–g.** She rolls the Swiss ball around her back, a movement which helps to achieve functional range for self care. **h.** Leaning against the ball, which is positioned between the patient and wall, she practices shoulder abduction, external rotation, and extension of the spine. **i.** The patient rotates her trunk under the stable shoulder girdle (horizontal abduction) of the right shoulder. **j.** Supporting herself from the forearms reduces the probability of making an evasive movement. The patient moves the proximal lever and the pivot point. The distal fixed point, the elbow, rests on the floor. **k.** Lying supine on the Swiss ball is a good position to allow gravity to assist forward flexion of the upper extremity.

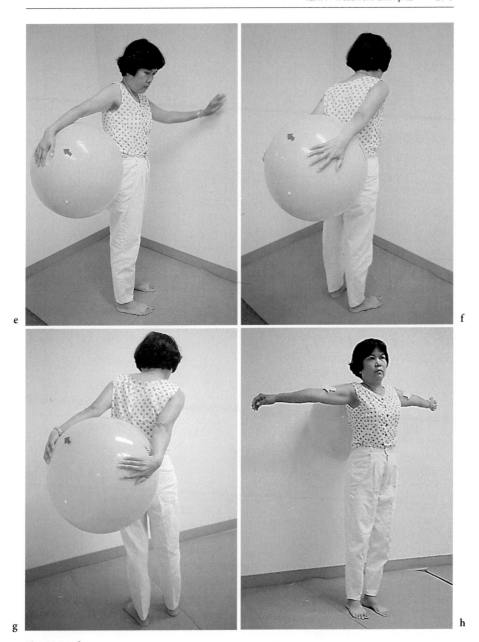

e

f

g

h

Fig. 12.1 e–h.

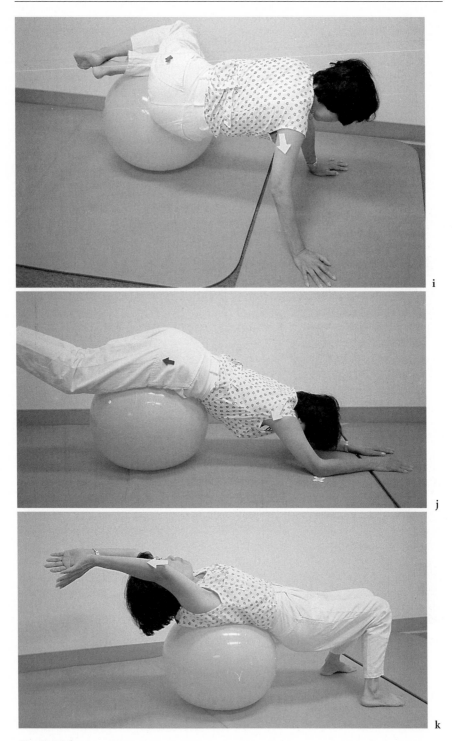

Fig. 12.1 i–k.

c). The patient adds rotation from the proximal lever (the trunk and scapula) by sitting on the right side of her knees (d; see the description of movement possibilities in Sect. 5.7).

Panels e–g. She rolls the Swiss ball around her back, a movement which helps achieve functional range for self-care. This exercise should be performed in both directions around the trunk.

Panel h. Leaning against the ball which is positioned between the patient and the wall, shoulder abduction, and extension and rotation of the spine can be practiced.

Panel i. The patient rotates her trunk under the stable shoulder girdle, which is a horizontal abduction of the right shoulder performed from the proximal lever.

Panel j. By supporting herself on her forearms, there is less possibility of making an evasive movement. The patient moves the proximal lever and the pivot point; the distal fixed point, the elbow, rests on the floor. This position is also helpful in treating patients who have difficulty supporting the weight of the body on their wrists.

Panel k. Forward flexion of the upper extremity with gravity assisting the movement can be performed lying supine on the Swiss ball. In this panel the patient assists the movement with her left arm. Notice that the patient is using a large base of support (keeping the feet wide apart) to maintain stability when moving.

The therapist can also stand behind the patient, hold on to her wrists, and let the patient gently pull her buttocks toward her heels. ROM of forward flexion increases because the patient pulls from the proximal lever. The wrists are the fixed points (Fig. 6.5).

Of course, in addition to these Swiss ball exercises there are many other treatment possibilities, one of which is to mobilize the patient's scapula manually. Other programs include aerobic activities to help patients regain a sense of control over their lives (Miller 1992). Proprioceptive neuromuscular facilitation is a good treatment using arm and scapular patterns (Voss et al. 1985; Adler et al. 1993). Other patients may benefit from the Feldenkrais approach, which increases "awareness through movement" (Feldenkrais 1972; Nelson 1989). Foam roll exercises (Parker 1992) can be performed in combination with the Swiss ball, and the patient can also use the Sitfit and other assistive devices as described in Chapter 8. Klein-Vogelbach (1991) offers a variety of therapeutic exercises that can be applied to these patients. All these concepts suggest exercises which can serve as examples, but many others can be also be used.

The advantage of using the Swiss ball as part of the treatment are:
- The possibility of exercising at home and monitoring the progress.
- The ability to combine proprioceptive and balance training with mobilization of joints, soft tissue and neural tissue in combination with strengthening exercises.
- Greater compliance in following a home program, because exercising is fun.
- The therapist can use her time for other treatment approaches and only readjust the patient's home program.

After Abdominal Surgery

A recent patient had spent several months in the hospital after life-threatening pancreatitis. He was unable to extend his fingers fully and lacked shoulder forward flexion and trunk extension. "It is amazing," he said, "I only had surgery to my stomach, yet I still have all these movement restrictions 11 months after the initial onset of the pancreatitis." This statement demonstrates a fact which is often overlooked by both patients and physicians.

Movement restrictions may remain many months after surgery or severe illness, and unless treated, the patient may never regain his movement potential. The patient could even develop new problems secondary to the acquired postural deficit.

 Figure 12.2a, b. A previously healthy 17-year-old man suffered severe abdominal injuries and a collapsed lung in a motor vehicle accident. He spent weeks in intensive care and suffered a weight loss of 30–40 lbs. Approximately 4 weeks after surgery the family requested physical therapy because of the patient's poor posture and general weakness. Panel a. The patient is unable to stand erect.
Panel b. Approximately 4 months after physical therapy treatments began, the patient's posture has improved considerably; he has gained weight and returned to school. According to the family, 14 months after the motor vehicle accident the patient was doing well, majoring in physical therapy, and excelling over classmates in racquet ball.

This patient is presented as an example throughout this volume. Figures 2.6 and 6.5 illustrate mobilization of the spine.

It is hypothetical but possible that gentle mobilization of the spine in all planes help to normalize parasympathetic and sympathetic (and therefore also autonomous) regulation, which may be affected after major abdominal injuries to the viscera.

Butler (1994) describes the following features of sympathetic pain pattern in greater detail.

Sympathetic pain patterns:
- Altered blood flow (reflected in red, white, or mottled skin color)
- Altered sweating
- Swelling or sensation of swelling
- Trophic changes (e.g., glossy skin)
- Abdominal bloating
- Pain/stiffness in the thoracic region
- Thoracic posture, such as forward head
- Patient complaints of pain or stiffness without the other signs above

---

The sympathetic slump can be defined as mechanical stimulation of the sympathetic trunk which results in altered peripheral sympathetic nervous system function and/or target tissue sensitivity (Slater et al. 1994; an adaptation of the sympathetic slump is presented in Fig. 2.6b).

Examples for the evaluation and treatment of these patients are presented in the figures of previous chapters:
- Figure 7.14a. The patient is unable to extend the trunk (secondary to general weakness).
- Figure 7.14b. The patient demonstrates the strength that he gained during six treatments. He is able to extend the trunk against gravity, with the arms in the midfrontal plane.
- Figure 7.16. Lack of trunk extension.
- Figures 8.20, 8.21. Foam roll exercises and soft tissue mobilization.

EXAMPLES

Figure 12.2c,d. Initially the goals of physical therapy for this patient were to mobilize the spine gently in all planes and increase the elasticity of the soft tissue. General conditioning and strengthening was also included in the exercise program. This highly motivated patient was given a 65-cm Swiss ball for home exercises.

Panel c. He also practiced squatting while working on the postural alignment of the trunk while standing and leaning against the wall to strengthen his lower extremities.

Panel d. In a second therapy session Thera-Band, sitfit, and foam roll exercises were added to the home program. The next three physical therapy treatments focused on coaching and teaching the patient on how to monitor himself and use gym equipment safely when working out. Reconditioning was the emphasis of this treatment.

The patient returned for a final, sixth visit approximately 4 months after treatment was initiated. By that time his strength, endurance, and mobility

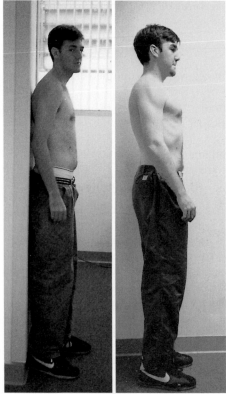

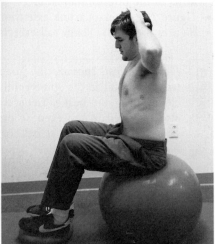

a

b

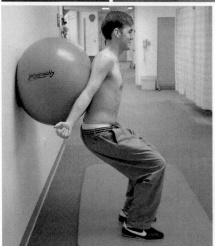

c

d

Fig. 12.2 a. Four weeks after a motor vehicle accident, total abdominal surgery, and a collapsed lung, the patient is unable to stand erect (first treatment session). **b.** Approximately 4 months after the first treatment and after six physical therapy sessions, the patient can stand erect. **c.** The patient mobilizes his back into extension while strengthening his quadriceps muscles. **d.** At the final visit (approximately 5 months after the accident), the patient demonstrates good upright posture of the trunk, good balance, and proprioception.

had improved considerably. The patient had good strength, skill, balance, and proprioception (Fig. 12.2 b, d).

12.2 Medical Patients

There are many medical conditions for which the Swiss ball can be used.

> The goal may be to reduce the weight of a body segment or part thereof if the patient needs to exercise and is very weak.

This could be the case in patients following cardiopulmonary conditions and after a prolonged illness such as pancreatitis, leukemia, cancer, and AIDS.

Exercising remains important for most patients to improve their cardio-vascular system and to avoid pneumonia, thrombosis, and other complications. Exercises can also help the patient to remain independent as long as possible (see also Chapters 2, 4, 10). At times the treatment may be palliative but nevertheless provide the patient with dignity and a feeling of worth. Attaining the highest level of physical and mental fitness may be an important factor in maintaining "wellness" (Toot 1992; Snyder 1992a,b). The therapist must meet the patient with understanding and a thorough knowledge of the surrounding issues, and interact well with other health care providers. Exercises which may be appropriate are described in Chapter 10 and can be adjusted to the patient's abilities and needs.

Because osteoporosis and ankylosing spondylitis are medical conditions which require particular attention, they serve here as treatment examples. Most of these exercises can also be applied to other medical conditions.

12.3 Osteoporosis

12.3.1 Introduction

Osteoporosis is a medical condition which lends itself well to the use of the Swiss ball. There are a few diseases in which osteoporosis occurs at an earlier age, but the treatment here is the same as described in this chapter. Type I osteoporosis in adults affects postmenopausal women, while type II is age-related and affects both men and women over the age of 70 – albeit women twice as frequently (Shipp 1993). Controlling pain and restoring confidence in mobility are the first of many steps in treating patients with osteoporosis (Shipp 1993). Without confidence when moving about, the patient becomes sedentary. This can lead to decreased bone density and increases the danger of falling because of the lack of strength, coordination, and balance. Most patients with advanced osteoporosis break their bones when falling. Pain is a part of this vicious cycle as it causes patients to be inactive when they actu-

EXAMPLES

Figure 12.3. Panel a. The kyphosis of the thoracic spine is apparent as the patient leans against the ball with her arms extending toward her back as far as possible without straining *(no forced movements!).* An insecure patient can use a PhysioRoll. Trying to lift the head (or one or both arms) in good alignment off the ball strengthens the neck and upper back extensors.

Panel b. The patient supports her chest on the ball while attempting to move the supinated and flexed arms with external rotation into the midfrontal plane. The movement is against gravity and the ball requires stabilization of all trunk muscles. The exercise can also be done with the patient sitting on a chair and leaning against a big ball positioned between her and the wall. The exercise is easier when sitting in a more vertical position than when kneeling, as demonstrated (put a pillow under the knees if the patient feels uncomfortable kneeling on the mat), because the lever which needs to be lifted against gravity is shorter.

Panel c. The patient demonstrates the second phase of the exercise "Donkey Stretch Yourself " (Sect. 9.4). This exercise can be used to promote extension of the spine with the assistance of gravity. The patient is able to do this exercise because she has good balance. At home the exercise can be performed more safely beside a sofa or between chairs that the patient can hold onto. Pillows can be placed under the head or lumbar spine to increase the diameter of the surface.

Figure 12.4. Thera-Band is used in combination with the Swiss ball. All exercises here promote postural alignment in combination with strengthening of the trunk muscles. The Swiss ball adds the element of support and at the same time requires muscles to stabilize because of the ball's mobility. Thera-Band adds resistance to the extremity muscles. The strength of the Thera-Band must match the patient's muscle strength.

 The exercise "Donkey Stretch Yourself " is not recommended for patients who may lose their balance!

All exercises which require movement in the sagittal plane can be performed on the PhysioRoll when first being learned. Many of the exercises described in Chapter 9 and illustrated throughout this volume can also be done if they meet the patient's and the therapist's goals and are adapted to the patient's ability. Bouncing gently when sitting in a good upright posture can enhance proprioceptive training and physiological compression to the spine (see the "Cowboy," Sect. 9.1).

Patients with osteoporosis who are unable to sit on a Swiss ball or do the exercises described above can work on strength, balance, and coordination

The management principles of physiotherapy in AS are described by Viitanen and Suni (1995), who give a thorough review of all systems affected by
the disease. Inner organs are sometimes also involved. Due to the activation
of inflammatory cells, common signs in AS include atrophy of the muscles
and skin and osteoporosis associated with fatigue (Viitanen and Suni 1995).

> Symptoms of fatigue are often ignored although fatigue ranks before
> pain in many patients who consider stiffness as their main problem
> (Calin et al. 1993).

Patients with AS often have back pain of at least 3 month's duration and frequently suffer from sacroiliitis. Peripheral joint manifestations can occur at
the hips and shoulders. Since the disease involves the enthesis, where ligaments attach to bone, the Achilles tendon can be affected as well (Reid
1996).

The disease is often diagnosed after radiographs indicate sacroiliac joint
or spinal fusion.

The antigen HL-A W27 is present in 95% of patients suffering from AS;
however, only about 20% of patients who have the antigen develop the disease. The male-female ratio has been estimated at 10:1 (Calin and Fries
1975). Recent studies confirm that women are affected more frequently at a
ratio of 2.5 to 1 in favour of men, but with a number of distinguishing features. The diagnosis is usually delayed in women, the progression less rapid
than in men, and the extent less severe than in men; in addition, subsequent
peripheral joint diseases and osteitis pubis is more common in women than
in men (Calin 1993).

There is a genetic component to AS. For example, several years ago a patient presented with the typical stooped posture of AS. A physical therapy
student was shown that the patient, sitting in the waiting room, could easily
be recognized as a "typical" AS patient. When the patient's name was called,
to the amazement of the therapist another patient, sitting beside the presumed AS patient, stood up. The therapist was puzzled at first because the
patient who reported did not appear ankylotic. The bafflement was cleared
up, however, when the patient asked the therapist whether his brother, who
was waiting outside and also suffered from AS, could participate in the treatment session. This proved to be the severely ankylotic man who had been
observed in the waiting room. It turned out that this severely ankylotic man
had encouraged his younger brother to attend therapy early because several
brothers of the same family had already suffered from AS.

To manage their disease AS patients usually receive nonsteroidal anti-inflammatory drugs and, most importantly, are encouraged to follow a program of regular exercise (Viitanen and Suni 1995). The importance of rigor-
ous physical therapy to improve and maintain mobility has been demonstrated in studies on the effects of comprehensive home physiotherapy
(Kraag et al. 1994) and the cost effectiveness of group physical therapy with

AS patients (Bakker et al. 1994). Although the additional cost for the beneficial effect of group therapy was calculated at U.S. $409 per patient per year (Bakker et al. 1994), this may be a minor cost because the long-term benefit may be much greater when quality-of-life improvements are considered. In the study, patients also received 3 hours of therapy (exercises, sport, and hydrotherapy). The cost would probably have been much lower if, for example, the patient had received only exercises and then attended a group sport activity such as volleyball or badminton.

In the author's experience, AS patients are generally highly motivated and very cooperative.

> Group activities also help patients socially to deal with their impairment; they learn that they are not alone, and that stiffness, fatigue, and pain are problems which all of them must deal with on a daily basis.

12.4.2 Treatment Approach

Evaluation

- The hamstrings and hip flexor muscles are frequently shortened as a result of the patient flexing his knees and hips to help balance the stiff spine.
- Posterior tilt of the pelvis and decreased lumbar lordosis can be expected in many AS patients who do not exercise.
- Stiffness of the thoracic spine and the costovertebral joints not only decreases the ability to expand the chest when breathing but also limits forward flexion of the arms in the shoulder joints.
- Patients often have a forward head posture.
- Patients suffer from muscle soreness and weakness.
- Osteoporosis may be present and associated with feeling of fatigue.

Treatment Goals

- Maintain good posture.
- Keep trunk and extremities as strong as possible.
- Keep spine as mobile as possible to prevent spine and hip joints fused in flexion.
- Maintain good mobility of the rib cage.
- Maintain good vital capacity.
- Establish independence in a home exercise program.
- Achieve the ability to participate in functional activities.

Only if these goals are achieved, can the patient remain functionally independent.

Treatment Plan

- Strengthening exercises to achieve and maintain the best possible erect posture
- Gentle mobilization of tight structures (soft tissue, muscles, neural tissues, and joints)
- Mobilization of the rib cage
- Breathing exercises
- Increased/maintained balance and coordination (fall prevention)
- Independence in home exercises
- Participation in sports activities

Precautions

- Patients suffering from AS frequently have a high tolerance to pain. Hunter and Dubo (1983) report a case of a patient who had suffered a cervical fracture following a fall down five steps who went duck hunting for 6 days before reporting to the physician.
- Fractures complicate AS and are often due to a minor fall (Hunter and Dubo 1983). The authors attribute this in some cases to partial or complete ankylosis of the hips. The fractures most commonly occur in the cervical region.
- Because of the limited ROM, weakness, and stiffness the patient can lose his balance easily.
- Avoid contact sports. Modify sports such as volleyball to improve safety and select patients carefully who qualify.
- Use a rather large Swiss ball (at least 65 cm diameter) for exercises to accommodate the decreased ROM of the spine, hips, and shoulders. Pillows behind the neck or low back may help accommodate the stiff spine.
- Be careful when the patient is in a more acute inflammatory phase.

Contraindications

- **Do not mobilize fused joints.**
- **Do not mobilize the hypermobile neck.**

12.4.3 Physical Therapy

Patients with AS should exercise daily.

They can benefit from swimming and aquatic exercises if the disease is not too advanced, and their balance is good. Participation in aerobic sports, such as cross-country skiing and volleyball, can be beneficial, but certain precautions should be taken. In patients with more advanced AS, sports which involve the risk of falling are contraindicated (Lindner 1989; Vom Bruch 1991). Manual therapy (Schauer 1989) is often appreciated by patients whose joints are tight but not fused. The author uses mobilization techniques described by Klein-Vogelbach (1991) for the thoracic spine and costovertebral joints. Patients report that these help them to breathe more easily because the ribs and thoracic spine feel less tight. Plüss (1989) describes a treatment based on Klein-Vogelbach's functional kinetics approach. Göhring (1989) demonstrates how breathing exercises can help the patient to increase the vital capacity by exercising.

Any therapy which increases mobility and strength of the spine and the extremities can be performed if precautions are observed.

12.4.4 Swiss Ball Exercises in AS

The ball is a functional tool because of its versatility. It combines mobilization of muscles, soft tissue, and neural tissue with strengthening exercises and balance training. Increased flexibility of the spine (combination of trunk rotation and side bending) can be achieved if the spine is not fused.

All the exercises demonstrated in this chapter may apply to patients with AS, depending on the severity of the disease. The PhysioRoll is useful when the patient is insecure and to mobilize lateral flexion of the spine (see Fig. 11.23). Exercises using the foam roll can be helpful for self-mobilization of a tight spine (see Sect. 8.2; Fig. 8.21).

Patients with AS do well in a group. Swiss ball exercises that can be performed with such a group are described in Sect. 13.5.1, Figs. 13.1–13.9. Both patient groups need to maintain or increase mobility of the spine and rib cage and emphasize extension of the spine. Breathing exercises should be included when exercising either group. Of course, there are many other patients who may benefit from such exercises, especially when mobility, balance, and strength of the trunk are the goal of the treatment.

References

Adler SS, Beckers D, Buck M (1993) PNF in practice. Springer, Berlin Heidelberg New York
Bakker C, Hidding A, van der Linden S, van Doorslaer E (1994) Cost effectiveness of group physical therapy compared to individualized therapy for ankylosing spondylitis. A randomized controlled trial. J Rheumatol 21:264–268
Bold RM, Grossmann A (1978) Stemmführung nach Brunkow. Enke Stuttgart
Brügger A (1990) Gesunde Körperhaltung im Alltag, 3rd edn. Brügger, Zürich
Butler DS (1994) The upper limb tension test revisited, 2nd edn. In: Grant R (ed) Physical therapy of the cervical and thoracic spine. Churchill Livingstone, New York
Calin A (1993) Ankylosing spondylitis. In: Maddison PJ, Isenberg DA, Woo P, Glass DN (eds) Oxford textbook of rheumatology. Oxford University Press, Oxford, pp 681–690

Calin A, Fries JF (1975) Striking prevalence of ankylosing spondylitis in "healthy" W27 positive males and females. N Engl J Med 293(17):835–839

Calin A, Edmunds L, Kennedy G (1993) Fatigue in ankylosing spondylitis – why it is ignored? J Rheumatol 20(6):991–995

Carrière B (1988) Edema: its development and treatment using lymph drainage massage. Clin Manage Phys Ther 8(5):19–21

Cyriax J (1982) Textbook of orthopaedic medicine, 8th edn. Baillière Tindall, London

Dannbeck S, Auer C (1996) Osteoporose: Therapiekonzept zur Vermeidung von Stürzen. Krankengymnastik 48 (3):358–366

Duncan PW, Lotze MT, Gerber LH, Rosenberg SA (1983) Incidence, recovery, and management of serratus anterior muscle palsy after axillary node dissection. Phys Ther 63(8):1243–1247

Feldenkrais M (1972) Awareness through movement. Harper & Row, New York

Flynn TW (1996) The thoracic spine and rib cage. Butterworth-Heinemann Boston

Göhring H (1989) Krakengymnastische Möglichkeiten zur Verbesserung und Erhaltung der Thoraxbeweglichkeit und der Atembewegung bei Morbus Bechterew. Krankengymnastik 41(1):47–53

Gutman H, Kersz T, Barzilai T, Haddad M, Reiss R (1990) Achievements of physical therapy in patients after modified radical mastectomy compared with quadrantectomy, axillary dissection, and radiation for carcinoma of the breast. Arch Surg 125:389–391

Hunter T, Dubo HIC (1983) Spinal fractures complicating ankylosing spondylitis. Arthritis Rheumat 26(6):751–759

Klein-Vogelbach S (1990) Ballgymnastik zur funktionellen Bewegungslehre, 3rd edn. Springer, Berlin Heidelberg New York

Klein-Vogelbach S (1991) Therapeutic exercises in functional kinetics. Springer, Berlin Heidelberg New York

Kraag G, Stokes B, Groh J, Helewa A, Goldsmith CH (1994) The effects of comprehensive home physiotherapy and supervision on patients with ankylosing spondylitis – an 8-month followup. J Rheumatol 21:261–263

Lindner W (1989) Gruppentherapie und Sport mit Bechterew Patienten. Krankengymnastik 41(1):14–19

List M (1996) Krankengymnastische Behandlung in der Traumatologie, 3rd edn. Springer, Berlin Heidelberg New York

Miller LT (1992) Postsurgry breast cancer outpatient program. Clin Manage Phys Ther 12(4):50–56

Nelson SH (1989) Playing with the entire self: the Feldenkrais method and musicians. Semin Neurol 9(2):97–104

Parker I (1992) Beyond conventional exercises. Phys Ther Forum 7:4–7

Plüss A-G (1989) Funktionelles Rückenmuskeltraining bei Morbus Bechterew. Krankengymnastik 41(1):38–46

Preisinger E, Wernhardt R (1996) Osteoporoseprävention – ein Übungsprogramm für Frauen nach der Menopause. Krankengymnastik 48(3):344–356

Reid ME (1996) Bone trauma and disease of the thoracic spine and ribs. In: Flynn TW (1996) The thoracic spine and rib cage. Butterworth-Heinemann, Boston, pp 87–105

Ritson F, Scott S (1996) Physiotherapy for osteoporosis. Physiotherapy 82(7):390–394

Rutherford OM (1990) The role of exercise in prevention of osteoporosis. Physiotherapy 76(9):522–526

Schauer U (1989) Spezifische Mobilisation bei Morbus Bechterew (manuelle Therapie). Krankengymnastik 41(1):25–30

Shipp KM (1993) To manage fragility. Phys Ther 1(10):70–75 and 98–100

Slater H, Vicenzino B, Wright A (1994) 'Sympathetic slump': the effects of a novel manual therapy technique on peripheral sympathetic nervous system function. J Manual Manipulative Ther 2(4):156–162

Snyder R (1992a) Coping: you and your patient with cancer. Clin Manage Phys Ther 12(4):64–69

Snyder R (1992b) Physical therapy in terminal illness. Clin Manage Phys Ther 12(4):96–100

Toot JL (1992) Tapestry of care. Clin Manage Phys Ther 12(4):9–10

Travell JG, Simons DG (1983) Myofascial pain and dysfunction: the trigger point manual. Williams & Wilkins, Baltimore

Travell JG, Simons DG (1992) Myofascial pain and dysfunction: the trigger point manual, vol 2. Williams & Wilkins, Baltimore

Umphred DA (ed) (1995) Neurological rehabilitation, 3rd edn. Mosby, St. Louis

Viitanen JV, Suni J (1995) Management principles of physiotherapy in ankylosing spondylitis – which treatments are effective. Physiotherapy 81(6):322–329

Vom Bruch H (1991) Sporttherapie bei Spondylitis ankylosans (Morbus Bechterew) unter besonderer Berücksichtigung des Volleyballspiels. Krankengymnastik 43(4):340–345 (I), 5:475–480 (II), 6:577–588 (III), 7:718–727 (IV)

Voss DE, Ionta MK, Myers BJ (1985) Proprioceptive neuromuscular facilitation, 3rd edn. Harper & Row, New York

Woods EN (1996) Managing and preventing osteoporosis Phys Ther 4(5):40–46

13 Neurological Outpatient Care

OBJECTIVES

By the end of this chapter the patient will be able to:
- Understand why and how the Swiss ball can be used for evaluation and treatment of neurological outpatients
- Find applications for Swiss ball exercises with patients of Parkinson's disease
- Use the Swiss ball to treat patients with hemiplegia
- Select exercises for patients suffering from multiple sclerosis
- Understand proprioceptive training in patients with muscular dystrophy
- Use the Swiss ball to treat children with neurological problems

13.1 Introduction

The field of neurology encompasses a great variety of diseases and injuries which can afflict any part of the central nervous system (CNS) or peripheral nervous system (PNS). It includes not only genetic diseases such as muscular dystrophy (MD) and some forms of cerebral palsy (CP), but also illnesses with unknown origin and gradual onset such as multiple sclerosis (MS), Parkinson's, Alzheimer's, and other degenerative diseases such as cerebellar atrophy. Tumors can also have an insidious onset and can cause severe neurological deficits. Other neurological conditions appear suddenly, triggered by an internal event, for example, a stroke caused by an embolus, hemorrhage, or ischemic event. Neurological problems can also arise as a consequence of infection or autoimmune reaction. Guillain-Barré syndrome expresses itself in the PNS, while metabolic diseases such as alcoholism can affect the basal ganglia, and metastasis from cancer can cause great damage to the brain or spinal cord. Injuries to the CNS or PNS can stem from external events and result in traumatic brain injury and/or spinal cord injury. Frequently these are the consequence of gun shots, stab wounds, or accidents. Complications at birth can cause CNS or PNS injuries (e.g., CP and Erb's palsy).

13.2 Symptoms

All areas of the nervous system can be affected (see also Chapter 2). Damage may be predominantly in one area (e.g., Parkinson's disease), involve the entire CNS (e.g., MS), or be limited to the PNS (e.g., Guillain-Barré syndrome).

The symptoms indicate which areas of the CNS or PNS are affected and to what extent, and these should guide the physician in making the medical diagnosis. The patient's specific disabilities and impairments should match the medical diagnosis if the latter reflects the state of the entire nervous system. Examples are presented below.

13.2.1 Cerebellar Injuries

Typical and Possible Symptoms

The cerebellum receives sensory input from the periphery and motor output from the cortex (Urbscheit and Oremland 1995). The cerebellum may act as an adaptive feedforward control system which programs or models voluntary movement skills based on a memory of previous sensory input and motor output (Ito 1970). The ability of motor imagery is also attributed to the cerebellum. The cerebellum and its connectors regulate muscle tone, and it relies on input from proprioceptive and vestibular as well as higher-center regulatory mechanisms (Umphred 1995).

Cerebellar damage can cause movement disorders, with the following associations on the same side of the lesion:
- Low muscle tone (hypotonicity)
- Muscle weakness up to 50% (asthenia)
- Lack of coordination (ataxia) of trunk and/or extremities
- Difficulty estimating a movement goal precisely (dysmetria; patients tend to over- or undershoot the aim)
- Problems with timing of rapid movements (dysdiadochkinesia)
- Difficulty translating the time and sequence of a simple movement into a smooth one (movement decomposition)
- Staggering gait

The patients may also have balance, speech (dysarthria), and voice problems (little modulation). Some patients have a tremor; this differs from the tremor in Parkinson's disease: cerebellar tremor has a higher frequency and disappears when the motor system is not running intentional programs. Problems can also occur in controlling eye movements (e.g., deviation to the contralateral side, nystagmus; Urbscheit and Oremland 1995).

Deficits in other systems, such as decreased proprioception and injuries to areas of the cortex, compound the problem because if the cerebellum does not obtain the correct input, its output is affected accordingly.

Most therapists have observed patients who manifest a number of these symptoms, any of which can be severely disabling.

A young dentist was diagnosed with MS. The patient had dysmetria, balance deficits, speech problems, and staggering gait. Unfortunately, others did not hesitate to make uninvited and inappropriate remarks about his evident intoxication so early in the day, when in fact he was merely trying to maintain his independence and gait.

Treatment Possibilities

The Swiss ball can be used with cerebellar injuries to:
- Increase muscle tonus [via increased proprioceptive input e.g., the "Cowboy" (Sect. 9.1), "Swing" (9.10), "Salamander" (9.9)]
- Strengthen muscles (e.g., the bridging exercise "Figurehead" (Sect. 9.18)]
- Develop coordination of trunk and extremities [e.g., midline orientation, alignment exercises such as the "Cowboy" (Sect. 9.1), "Perpetual Motion" (9.22), "Dolphin" (9.29), "Cocktail Party" (9.28), "Scissors" (9.19)]
- Develop movement precision, speed, coordination, and smoothness [e.g., "Perpetual Motion" (Sect. 9.22), "Swing" (9.10), "Crab" (9.12)]
- Perform pregait training by working on submovements (or components of gait) such as alternate leg movements, alignment while moving, and gait speed [e.g., "Perpetual Motion" (Sect. 9.22), "Cowboy" (9.1), "Scale" (9.2)]
- Increase balance [various exercises with the patient sitting on the ball, e.g., "Cowboy" (Sect. 9.1), "Scale" (9.2), "Cocktail Party" (9.28), "Dolphin" (9.29)]

Evaluation of Submovements

Any complex movement is a composition of a number of submovements. For example, walking involves a sequence of movements which enable the person to take even-length steps, in a straight line, and at a certain speed while maintaining the trunk in an erect posture and swinging the arms alternatively (or in parallel if gait velocity is very slow). Each part of the movement sequence can be considered a submovement.

Evaluating submovements can reveal important details of the underlying motor process because the patient can make better use of the feedback information.

With increased practice a subject spends less time on corrective feedback-based secondary submovements which affect his ability to acquire and retain the skill needed to master the motor task (Abrams and Pratt 1993).

The Swiss ball can be used to evaluate and practice the entire range of submovements, including: moving an arm or a leg in a straight line, moving a limb at a certain speed, attempting to make movements smooth, and trying to center the body when sitting on the ball. The patient can take alternate steps (in the same spot) when bouncing on the ball and can practice swinging the arms while bouncing and balancing.

> At the end, after adding more and more submovements into a sequence, the patient should practice the entire movement sequence and finish with functional activities such as walking or balancing on a stable surface to benefit from the training.

This carryover into practice is crucial for therapeutic ball exercises to have a functional effect.

Evaluation of submovements on the "uninvolved" side can help the therapist determine whether the side is truly uninvolved, or to what extent it is part of the problem.

Disorders which affect primarily the basal ganglia, such as Parkinson's and Huntington's diseases, and those due to the effect of alcoholism differ from cerebellar injuries.

> Disorders of the basal ganglia manifest themselves in symptoms that vary depending on the disease but always result in disturbance of muscle tonus and affect involuntary movements (Melnick 1995).

Patients suffering from Parkinson's disease, for example, have difficulty with initiation and control of movement and posture.

13.2.2 Parkinson's Disease

Typical and Possible Symptoms

Typical and possible symptoms arising from damage to the basal ganglia in patients with Parkinson's disease:

- Lack of automatic movement (akinesia), bradykinesia, decreased movement
- Rigidity (cogwheel-type movement of extremities)
- Festinating gait (propulsion and/or retropulsion) with difficulty starting, stopping, and turning around
- Postural instability (probably due to symptoms described above, as well as decreased sensory processing)
- Tremor (4–7 beats per second), especially distally (hands), which continues at rest and decreases with movement
- Attention and learning deficits (especially declarative; these can occur at a later stage)

Because of the possible involvement of other important areas of the CNS, such as hypothalamus and the sympathetic nervous system, patients can also suffer from increased perspiration, dry skin (seborrhea), or oily skin.

Treatment Possibilities

The Swiss ball can be used with patients suffering from Parkinson's disease to:
- Trigger automatic movements by kicking, catching or throwing a ball
- Facilitate flexion/extension, ab- and adduction movements with the leg or arm on the ball (because the patient moves but does not lift the extremity in space when it is supported by a Swiss ball)
- Promote postural exercises, such as moving the spine in extension [e.g., "Figurehead" (Sect. 9.18), "Sea Gull" (9.6), "Donkey Stretch Yourself" (9.4)]
- Train postural alignment combined with balance training [e.g., "Cowboy" (Sect. 9.1)]
- Practice submovements (as described above)

13.2.3 Cerebral Vascular Accidents

Patients who have suffered a cerebral vascular accident (CVA), commonly known as "stroke," exhibit signs which depend greatly on the location in the brain or brain stem where the stroke occurred and on the extent of damage. Because the cerebral cortex maintains an "advice and consent" relationship with the basal ganglia and the cerebellum (Umphred 1995), damage to the cerebral cortex affects these areas as well. The deficits can appear within seconds, minutes, hours, or even a few days after the CVA, and the combination of the deficits enables the physician to detect both the location and the extent of the defect (Ryerson 1995).

Typical and Possible Symptoms

- Hemiplegia with low tone at onset and spasticity later
- Sensory deficits
- Visual field defects
- Aphasia (global, receptive, or expressive) and/or dysarthria
- Mental and intellectual impairment
- Lack of postural control

The patients may also have various other symptoms such as apraxia (perceptual difficulty in carrying out a movement), decreased sense of touch, vibration or position, and weakness of the vocal cords.

Although function on the contralateral side is usually more impaired, Jones et al. (1989) found that ipsilateral reaction time, speed, steadiness, steady movement, random tracking, step tracking, and combination of tracking were impaired throughout the 1-year follow-up period following a stroke. Smutok et al. (1989) also investigated unilateral brain damage and concluded that therapy for the nonhemiplegic side should be incorporated into comprehensive treatment programs because motor function can be affected adversely on the ipsilateral side.

Treatment Possibilities

The Swiss ball can be used in patients with hemiplegia to:

- Position the paralyzed limb so that the patient can observe passive or active movement (especially when the patient has visual field defects, dots may help the patient to attend to the task)
- Manage tone, by selecting movements which are fast and stimulating, or slow, rhythmic, and relaxing
- Practice dissociation of the limbs [e.g., as in the exercise "Perpetual Motion" (Sect. 9.22)] where one leg is flexed, the other extended, and alternate movement must be coordinated and timed)
- Practice submovements and movement sequences of pregait exercises (e.g., to learn to move the legs alternately, in good alignment, at a gait speed)
- Strengthen the lower or upper extremities to enable the weak patient to move a limb without having to lift it (promoting selective movements)
- Work on balance and trunk stabilization
- Learn proprioceptive training ["Cowboy" (Sect. 9.1), "Swing" (9.10), "Salamander" (9.9) and other exercises]

Although motor dysfunction (spasticity) is usually the most obvious sign in hemiplegia, sensory deficit and aphasia compound the problem. Occasionally they are the major problem.

> The ability of accurate, visually guided movement is a critical motor skill (Grafton et al. 1992). Therapists should be reminded to position the patient so that he can see the part of the body which is moved, or which he tries to move.

The patient may be helped to identify the body part and to concentrate on the task of moving by means of tactile (touching, rubbing, tapping) or visual attention (placing colored dots on the foot, knee or hand). The therapist should also allow the patient to process the information and give him time to visualize the planned movement and attempt to carry it out.

> **EXAMPLES**
>
> A patient whose greatest problem was that he had no sensory or kinesthetic awareness of his arm was able to walk and move his arms fairly well. One day he called his wife, claiming that someone was choking him. He was not aware that he was in fact choking himself with his "hemiplegic" hand.

13.2.4 Multiple Sclerosis

Typical and Possible Symptoms

MS is one of the least predictable neurological diseases. It can be very vicious in its progression and selection of areas in the brain and spinal cord. It can disable very young adults and cause grief, sadness, and frustration for the entire family. Patients may show signs of hemiplegia, paraplegia, quadriplegia, or monoplegia. Potential symptoms extend over a wide range, including spasticity, ataxia, tremor, weakness, sensory deficits, balance, vision, and bladder problems, often in aggravating combinations. Some patients have only a few attacks in their lifetime with only minor symptoms, and recover to their previous function, while others suffer frequent relapses, and still others experience continuous progression of the disease. Visual deficits and bladder problems are often associated with the first symptoms of MS. Patients fatigue easily and need rest periods when exercising.

> Energy conservation is very important.

Detailed information about the disease for therapists working with MS patients is provided by Frankel (1995).

Treatment Possibilities

All Swiss ball applications described in this chapter apply to MS patients. The findings of hemiplegia, balance problems, and paraplegia, for example, determine which exercises would be beneficial to the patient. The Swiss ball can also be used to:
- Teach the family to assist the patient with ROM and stretching exercises
- Maintain current muscle strength (efficient use of muscles)
- Combine movements for strength with balance and coordination
- Provide the patient with a home exercise program

As described above, cerebellar involvement is not uncommon in patients with MS. Therapists must reevaluate the patient after each relapse and continuously adapt the exercises to the new findings. The patient and family must be given emotional support and understanding to deal realistically with the disease. Social services should be involved if required.

13.3 Restoration of Function

The patient's general life-style, age, general condition, and attitude may influence the recovery or the speed of progression of a disease. The plasticity of the brain and behavioral factors contribute greatly to the restoration of lost function.

13.3.1 Plasticity of the Brain

Fortunately, new knowledge about the plasticity of the brain (see also Sect. 3.5) provides hope to many patients and therapists. Especially after an injury to the CNS, most patients are able to improve function over the subsequent 3–18 months, although paresis, sensory, and cognitive loss may remain the same. This is because spontaneous recovery may occur of reversibly edematous and metabolically depressed tissue. Strong motivation, a supportive milieu (as well as assistive devices), and compensatory behavioral training are also contributing factors. Dobkin (1993) attributes this to *"numerous parallel systems that cooperate to manage the diverse information necessary for the rapid, precise, and yet highly flexible control of multijoint movements. These circuits might contribute to spontaneous and training induced recovery of function."*

As any experienced neurological therapist can testify, some patients continue to recover many years after an injury to the CNS. Bach-Y-Rita (1987) depicts plasticity of the brain as its ability to unmask neural pathways and collateral sprouting from intact cells to denervated regions. The capacity of the CNS to modify organization and function assists the patient in recovery, for example, after a stroke. Brodal (1973) described in great detail his recovery after a stroke which left him paralyzed on his right side. He observed that *"scrutiny of the fiber connection of the CNS as a whole leaves one with the conviction that there are morphological possibilities for an impulse from a certain part of the brain to be transmitted along circumvential routes or varying complexity to virtual every other part of the CNS!"*

Specific forms of intervention can facilitate positive plasticity in the damaged brain. In recovery after a stroke or other brain injury, brain circuitry is capable of forming new connections well into old age (Winstein 1995).

In very young children the plasticity of the brain can help to assist motor programs to develop and improve function (e.g., in patients with CP).

> All major systems of the CNS are interlocking, codependent, and at no time stand isolated from one another; therefore their cooperation is very important in recovery or in trying to maintain functional independence as long as possible in a progressive disease affecting the CNS (Umphred 1995).

> Active participation and practice, together with meaningful goals, are behavioral factors that influence the plasticity/recovery of motor function (Winstein 1995). This is why the Swiss ball is a useful tool.

genuine stress incontinence by pelvic floor musculature exercises. They discovered that 14 patients who had achieved initial success after a supervised 4-week course in Kegel exercises had a disappointing result at 5-year follow-up.

> Surprisingly only 1 of 10 patients (who had responded) continued to exercise, while the others had ceased exercising because of lack of time or motivation.

Some authors suggest that the combination of biofeedback, electrical stimulation, or vaginal cones with Kegel exercises may enhance training in patients with genuine stress incontinence or an unstable bladder (McCandless and Mason 1995; McIntosh et al. 1993). Exercising the pelvic floor with artificial devices such as cones and electrical stimulation is clearly less functional.

> Motivation and enthusiastic instruction seems a crucial factor in the effectiveness of exercises (Bø et al. 1990; Henalla et al. 1988).

Tibæk (1994) also found improvement through pelvic floor exercises in patients with USI and mixed USI with urge incontinence, noting a relationship between the amount/intensity of treatment, good instruction, and result. Surprisingly, patients with moderate and severe incontinence demonstrated better results than those with mild USI; this may be due in part to greater motivation by patients with moderate or severe incontinence to perform daily exercises.

> It is important in the treatment to explain exercises and to use diagrams to locate the perineal muscles for patients.

However, this information alone is not sufficient. The therapist must instill a profound appreciation of how to activate the pelvic floor and of the functions that it has.

The studies discussed above generally point out the following:
- Kegel exercises are the most common pelvic floor muscle exercises in the United States.
- Physical therapists are seldom involved in treatment of USI in the United States. It is more common that nurses treat the patients, providing electrical stimulation and exercises.
- Motivation is a crucial factor in helping the patient to maintain the exercise routine and improve strength.
- Single treatments or handing out exercise sheets with explanations is not sufficient to improve the patient's problem.

- Treatment is more successful when patients are followed over several weeks or months.
- Patients benefit from group treatment.

> Physical therapists must rethink pelvic floor exercises and include exercises that are motivating and functional.

A recent study by Byl et al. (1997) investigated the role of isolated versus complex movements in primates. Although the goal of the study was to improve understanding of repetitive strain injuries to the hand, its results are probably relevant to muscular problems of the pelvic floor. The study concluded that isolated repetitive movements cause both substantial degradation of the hand representation in the anterior parietal cortex and motor deterioration, while more variable strategies cause only mild degradation of the hand representation in the anterior parietal cortex and preserve motor control.

This study may explain why an isolated repetitve movement such as squeezing the pelvic floor muscles 300 times per day does not in fact improve its function. Instead, it may provide insight into why the performance of isolated muscle training of the pelvic floor does not help to alleviate pain and the discomfort from many other pelvic floor dysfunctions. On the other hand, this paper supports the concept of linking pelvic floor strengthening exercises to such functional activities as are described in this chapter. These compare to variable strategies which may have a more benficial input to the somatosensory cortex than rigidly sterotyped exercises.

The Swiss ball is a tool which can be used for the retraining of weak pelvic floor muscles. The exercises are functional because they incorporate activity of the pulmonary diaphragm and the abdominal and back muscles with restoration of the pelvic floor, and can also be performed while watching television or holding a baby. Exercises following the Tanzberger concept are more fun to carry out than are the traditional Kegel exercises. However, it is of paramount importance that patients first learn and understand the exercises in depth and know and feel how to do them correctly before attempting to exercise independently.

14.2 Tanzberger Concept for Functional Exercises of the Pelvic Floor

The Swiss ball has become an indispensable tool and an ideal intermediary of movement for training the pelvic floor muscles. The Tanzberger (1991a,b, 1992, 1994) concept differs from Kegel exercises, electrical stimulation, and the use the of cones, all of which advocate isolated muscle contractures of primarily the pubococcygeus muscle.

> The goal of the Tanzberger concept is to restore the physiological activity of the pelvic floor/sphincter system.

To achieve this, very differentiated stimuli must be given to improve the strength to close urethra and anus, to improve the strength of the vaginal cuff, and to increase and activate the lifting strength (levator function) of the pelvic diaphragm.

> Since the pelvic floor is part of a compartment composed of the pulmonary diaphragm, abdominal, and back muscles, therapeutic exercises (with or without the Swiss ball) are based on the functional connection of the pelvic floor with the pulmonary diaphragm and the abdominal and back muscles.

This chapter presents the basic ideas of this concept for restoring the exit structures of the pelvis, selecting therapeutic exercises based on these functional connections.

14.3 Anatomy of the Pelvic Floor

14.3.1 The Three Layers of the Pelvic Floor

The pelvic floor consists of tissues that span the opening of the bony pelvis and provides support for the abdominal and pelvic viscera that rest upon it (Wall 1994). The pelvic floor is made up of three main supportive layers.

The first layer is the endopelvic fascia, a connective fibromuscular tissue consisting of collagen, elastin, smooth muscle, and visceral ligaments and fascia. It arises from the pelvic walls and inserts to the pelvic organs (uterus, cervix). The endopelvic fascia also supports the bladder neck and urethra, and the posterior attachment of the vagina prevents the rectum from prolapsing forward.

> The endopelvic fascia contains the autonomic nerves to the uterus and bladder. Endopelvic ligaments are oriented in a vertical direction and suspend the pelvic organs which are supported by the second layer, the pelvic diaphragm.

Suspension of the cardinal and uterosacral "ligaments" in a vertical direction makes sense when one considers the forces impacting the upright woman, rather than an anesthetized patient lying on an operating table (Wall 1994).

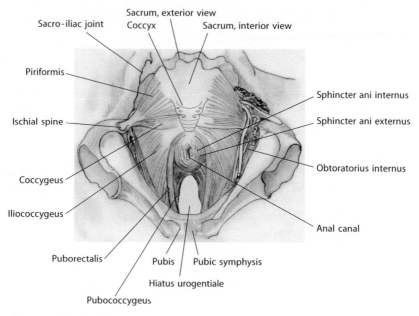

Fig. 14.1. Pelvic diaphragm. (Modified, from Testut 1948).

> Injuries to the first layer can cause failure to support the pelvic organs.

The second layer of the pelvic floor consists of the structure of the levator ani muscle (also known as puboviscera muscle), the coccygeus muscle, and their fascial covering. The broad muscle sling derives from the posterior surface of the superior rami of the pubis, the inner surface of the ischial spine, and the obturator fascia. The muscle fibers insert around the vagina and rectum, forming a functional sphincter for each, into the raphe in the midline between vagina and rectum, below the rectum and into the coccyx (Cunningham et al. 1993). The pubococcygeus, puborectalis, iliococcygeus (which supports the pelvic viscera), and coccygeus muscles are part of the levator ani muscle (Fig. 14.1).

> The muscle fibers of the pubococcygeus and puborectalis muscles run in a generally anterior/posterior direction and are part of the muscle sling. The fibers of the iliococcygeus and coccygeus muscles extend in a diagonal direction. During vaginal birth muscles of this layer can be injured and nerves damaged. This can cause decreased resting tonus and weakness.

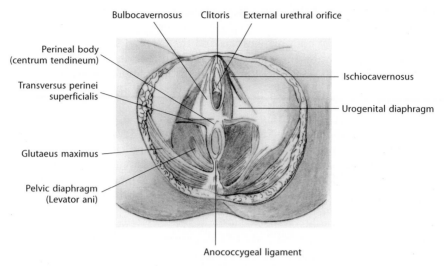

Bulbocavernosus   Clitoris   External urethral orifice

Perineal body
(centrum tendineum)

Transversus perinei
superficialis

Glutaeus maximus

Pelvic diaphragm
(Levator ani)

Ischiocavernosus

Urogenital diaphragm

Anococcygeal ligament

Fig. 14.2. Female urogenital diaphragm. (Modified, from Testut 1948).

The third layer, known as the urogenital diaphragm, lies external to the pelvic diaphragm. This perineal membrane which extends from the ischial tuberosities to the symphysis pubis is comprised of the deep transverse perineal and superficial perineal muscles, the fibers of which run in a frontal direction. The constrictor of the urethra and the external anal sphincter muscle form muscle slings, as does the bulbocavernosus muscle in women. In men it runs diagonally. The internal and external fascia coverings are also part of the urogenital diaphragm.

The perineal body consists of fibrous tissue between the vagina and the anus. It receives fibers from the bulbocavernosus, superficial transverse perineal, external anal sphincter muscles, and perineal membrane (Fig. 14.2). These structures support the perineum (pelvic and urogenital diaphragms).

> The perineal body is often torn or injured by incision during vaginal birth (Wall 1994; Cunningham et al. 1993; Adams and Frahm 1995).

14.3.2 Innervation of the Pelvic Floor Muscles

Neural stimulation of both diaphragms and the external sphincter muscles is supplied somatically by the pudendal nerve, which originates at the spinal cord at the level of S2–S4. The inner sphincter muscles are under autonomic control.

> The sympathetic nerve (arising at the level of T11–L2 of the spinal cord) is responsible for the phases of storage and closing of the bladder. The parasympathetic nerve is responsible for emptying and opening the bladder (Jäning 1995). To remember the innervation, Tanzberger uses the following mnemonic: "It is *sympathetic* to be *continent, parasympathetic* to *pee.*"

Continence requires that the detrusor muscle (the bladder) remain relaxed while the sphincter muscle contracts; during micturition (emptying of the bladder) the sphincter muscle must relax while the detrusor muscle contracts. Several neuronal mechanisms take part in regulating continence.

> In addition to the neural regulation of continence there is pontine control of bladder function. Since continence and micturition are also regulated by the brain stem, hypothalamus, and cortex, a person is able to "override" the urge to empty the bladder or can voluntarily empty it (Jäning 1995).

> Defecation and maintenance of bowel continence is regulated by the parasympathetic sacral, sympathetic thoracolumbar, and somatomotor mechanisms.

Defecation is supported by voluntary control and intra-abdominal pressure, tightening of abdominal muscles, and activity of the pulmonary diaphragm. Stretching of the rectum walls results in reflectory relaxation of the internal anal sphincter muscle (Jäning 1995).

14.3.3 Muscle Physiology of the Pelvic Floor

Both diaphragms (the caudal urogenital and the inner pelvic diaphragm) and the external sphincter muscles of the urethra and the rectum serve as a functional unit.

> It is important to realize that the striated levator ani muscles (pelvic diaphragm) consist of slow- and fast-twitch fibers while the external anal sphincter muscle has predominantly slow-twitch fibers (Bump et al. 1991); 70% of the fibers of the levator ani muscle are of the slow-twitch type while 30% are fast-twitch fibers (Wall et al. 1993).

The slow-twitch fibers maintain some constant involuntary tone of the levator ani muscle. The tone varies with posture and the person's alertness. The internal anal sphincter (which is under autonomic control) keeps the rectum closed during sleep.

> The external anal sphincter muscle cannot be contracted in isolation but is accompanied by general contractions of the perineal muscles, especially the sphincter urethrae.

Under conditions of stress, such as coughing or straining, the external (striated) urethral sphincter muscle is very active, while under normal conditions the internal vesical sphincter (smooth muscle) also maintains continence (Basmajian and Luca 1985).

> This knowledge must be applied when selecting stimulating exercises, which should always challenge the muscle function.

Bump et al. (1991) observe that "undoubtedly the resting tone of these slow-twitch fibers in the levator group is the important factor in keeping the levator hiatus essentially closed in patients with normal support."

> Providing verbal and visual instructions/explanations are important for the patient to understand the anatomy and physiology of the invisible pelvic floor.

14.4 The Pelvic Floor and its Functional Connections

14.4.1 Functions

Primary Function

The primary function of the pelvic floor is to achieve urinary and fecal continence, but it also must be able to relax to allow the expulsion of urine and feces. Continence is achieved by the intrinsic structures of the lower urinary tract and the rectum.

The following muscles are involved:
- The intrinsic structures (smooth muscles) of the lower urethra and colon
  - The internal urethral sphincter muscle with endopelvic fascia
  - The internal anal sphincter muscle and the connective tissue surrounding the anus (perineal body)
- The extrinsic striated diaphragms and the imbedded external sphincter muscles
  - Levator ani muscle
  - Perineal muscles
  - External urethrae and anal sphincter muscles

> Together these intrinsic and extrinsic muscles are responsible for continence of urine, gas, and feces, and they ensure the ability to store and empty the contents of (the storage organs) bladder and rectum.

Secondary Function

The secondary function is the true pelvic "floor" function. The pelvic floor achieves its function of supporting and holding in cooperation with the muscles of the abdominal compartment (Richter 1985).

In an upright posture the following muscles are part of the abdominal compartment:
- ventral: abdominal muscles
- rostral: pulmonary diaphragm
- dorsal: back muscles
- caudal: pelvic floor

These various muscle groups support the levator ani and sphincter muscle function by their functional connection with each other.

> During coughing, straining, jumping, or running, these muscles must work together to serve as support for the pelvic floor muscles.

14.4.2 Training Functional Connections of the Pelvic Floor to Thorax and Legs

The movement of the Swiss ball (especially in a sitting position) can be used to exercise simultaneously the various muscular structures described above as a functional unit with the pelvic floor. There is a functional relationship of movement between the body segments pelvis–legs and pelvis–thorax (Klein-Vogelbach 1990, 1991). Additional possibilities for stimulating physiological functions are present while breathing because the pulmonary diaphragm affects the pelvic diaphragm centrally (within the body). The rhythmic movement of breathing supports abdominal and pelvic floor muscle activity synergistically.

> During inhalation both abdominal and pelvic floor muscles support the downward movement of the pulmonary diaphragm while the pelvic floor swings into an upward direction during exhalation.

Any change in pressure during the costodiaphramatic mechanism affects not only the muscles of the abdominal wall but also the pelvic floor muscles reactively (Schmitt 1981).

> Guided stenotic exhalation (or straining) achieves activation not only of the diaphragm pulmonale but also the internal and external oblique abdominal muscles (Basmajian and De Luca 1985).

This results in a dynamic increase in tension (a reaction which can be felt) in the functional unit pelvic floor/sphincter. Therapeutic movement sequences that are natural, make sense, and are fun to carry out provide the patient an important motivation to continue exercising by himself.

> The success of the exercises is demonstrated by changes in the patient's symptoms.

Swiss ball exercises improve sensory awareness of the pelvic floor muscles with each movement. This promotes spontaneous acceptance of new exercises, which is also very self-motivating. The patients are encouraged to exercise daily at home.

Retraining of the pelvic floor is achieved through the characteristic properties of the ball with its unique spherical shape and elasticity, which compliments the spherical form of its contact with the ischial tuberosities. In a sitting position the contact of these two round forms with each other allows a unique communication and translation of the rolling movement while the pelvis continuously changes its positions in relationship to the ball. This enhances the perception and increases the muscle strength of the pelvic floor. Primary and secondary functions of the pelvic floor can be retrained with the Swiss ball. It can be used for pelvic floor exercises and training of sphincter muscles both for prevention and restoration.

14.5 Medical Conditions Which May Require Pelvic Floor Exercises

14.5.1 Gynecological Applications

During pregnancy and the preparation for delivery women can be instructed in pelvic floor exercises to prevent weakness of the pelvic floor muscles and to improve awareness of tension and relaxation in preparation for the delivery. During the opening contractures of delivery the goal of the exercises is to offset tension by means of movement. This can help prevent tensing up during delivery.

> **After childbirth pelvic floor exercises can be started on about the 12th day postpartum (phase of recovery).**

In the puerperium (first 6 weeks postpartum) the reproductive tract begins to return anatomically to a normal nonpregnant state, and ovulation is reestablished in most women who do not breastfeed.

> During this period the abdominal walls, which are soft and flabby, return to normal over a period of several weeks especially when aided by exercises (Cunningham et al. 1993).

Sometimes the muscles remain atonic and the abdominal wall lax. Obstetrical factors such as length of labor, infant head circumference, birthweight, and episiotomy are associated with stress incontinence after delivery.

> Pelvic nerve injuries sustained during childbirth can cause partially denervated muscles and result in gradual loss of pelvic tone (Wall 1994; Wall and Davidson 1992).

> The postpartum treatment goals in physical therapy are therefore to support of processes which help the body to return to its predelivery state and to increase the tone of the pelvic floor and abdominal muscles.

Exercising patients with gynecological problems, to train the pelvic floor individually or in small groups, can also help to prevent damage if they are educated in avoiding undue strain to the pelvic floor. Surgery can often be prevented or delayed in cases of minimal pathology, and surgical results postoperatively can be improved.

In patients who suffer from pelvic floor and sphincter insufficiency in connection with descending urogenitals and stress incontinence of urine, gas, and stool, the goal of the treatment is to achieve topographical improvement and continence.

14.5.2 Urological and Proctological Applications

> Incontinence and sphincter insufficiency are sometimes complications after radical prostatectomy (Fig. 14.3).

The goal of treatment in these cases is to achieve continence and sphincter sufficiency. Anal insufficiency of the sphincter muscle (Fig. 14.4) usually results in incontinence of gas and stool.

> The physical therapy goal is to build up elastic strength, achieve continence, and sufficiency of the sphincter muscle.

Patients affected by proctospasm and anism usually have difficulty in voluntarily relaxing the pelvic floor and sphincter muscles.

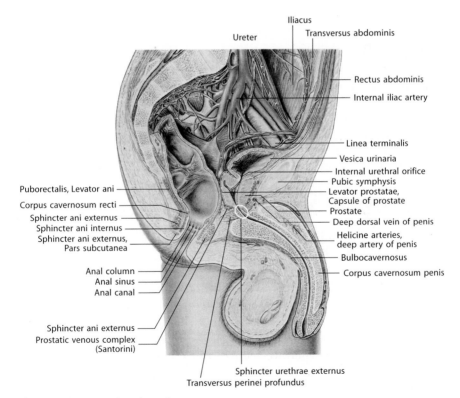

Fig. 14.3. Rectum and anal canal.

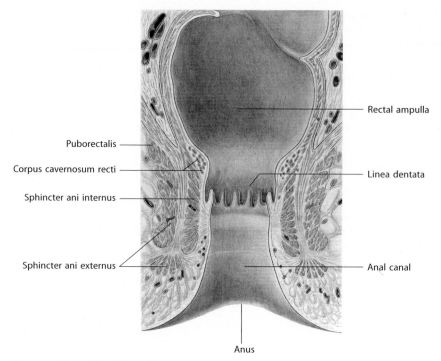

Puborectalis

Corpus cavernosum recti

Sphincter ani internus

Sphincter ani externus

Rectal ampulla

Linea dentata

Anal canal

Anus

Fig. 14.4. The pelvis of the male.

> The goals of physical therapy are to improve circulation and achieve balance of tension so that the patient can learn to relax the tight structures.

14.6 Retraining the Pelvic Floor Muscles

14.6.1 Preconditions for Functional Exercise of the Invisible Pelvic Floor Muscles

> Muscle activity of the pelvic floor is normally automatic and subconscious, operating on procedural synergetic programming.

The therapist must create the following three preconditions for the patient to be able voluntarily to influence muscle strength through exercises and acquire a conscious awareness of the pelvic floor:
- The patient must know the location and the extent of the pelvic floor muscles and be able to visualize their position.

- The patient must understand the function of the pelvic floor muscles.
- The patient must be able to accompany the changes of the muscles function with a concrete inner picture.

14.6.2 Treatment Considerations for Sphincter Muscle Weakness

EXAMPLES A patient suffering primarily from weakness of the sphincter muscle should be offered exercises which are appropriate for slow-twitch fibers to achieve external sphincter muscle control. These exercises must be in a slow, rhythmic movement which accompanies the flow of tension, gradually changing from increasing the tension, tightening, to letting go again and relaxing.

This physiological change should be synchronized with the rhythm of breathing: expiration while tightening, and inspiration while letting go of the tension – expiration, inspiration, etc.

EXAMPLES Figure 14.5. The exercise "Roll-On" illustrates how the slow-twitch fibers can be activated in an anterior-posterior direction. The exercise "Right Stop–Left Stop" helps to strengthen muscle fibers that run in a frontal direction.

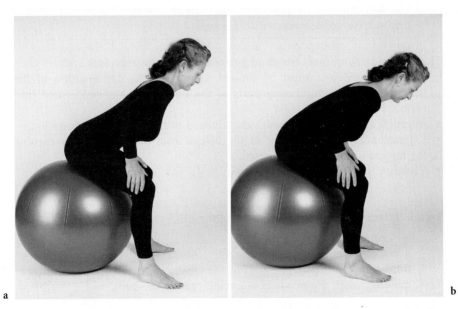

a   b

Fig. 14.5 a, b. "Roll-On" starting and end position. Exercise which trains urogenital diaphragm and urethra sphincter muscle. (Photographs by R. Tanzberger).

14.6.3 Treatment of Descending Diaphragm Pelvis with Gaping Urogenital Hiatus (Postpartum)

When the patient suffers from a descending diaphragm pelvis with a gaping urogenital hiatus after childbirth, it is recommended that the above rhythmic change in tension (while sitting on the Swiss ball rocking backward and forward) be supplemented by a functional stimulus for quick reaction of the fast-twitch fibers.

> This can be achieved with exercises that promote bouncing and are accompanied by short explosive words such as "kick and kick," or "hop and hop" which emphasize the rhythm of the movement and are stimulating. The exercise "Kick-and-Kick" (Fig. 14.11) stimulates principally fast-twitch fibers of the muscles of the pelvic diaphragm.

14.6.4 Performance and Sequence of Exercises for Treatment of Incontinence

The primary movement is the rolling movement at the contact between pelvis and ball. The primary movement intensifies the muscle activity of the pelvic floor under certain conditions and limitations.

> The ball must be inflated to firmness to ensure that the ischial tuberosities have good contact with the ball.

The necessary conditions for good performance of the exercises are:
- The ball movement must be limited to prevent the continuation of the movement to the connecting parts of the body (legs and ankle, and thoracic spine).
- Alternate rhythmic movements are adjusted to the phases of respiration.
- Expiration against resistance of the lips or roof of the palate by turning the tongue upward and backward.
- Visualization of the muscular activity.

14.6.5 Effect of the Bouncing Movement

> Bouncing and hopping on the ball provoke reactive muscle contractions in both diaphragms and in the closing structures (the sphincter muscles, when the pelvis is bouncing against the ball).

This can be used as a test of continence because the bouncing movement moves the visceral content, and with its weight it stimulates the levator ani muscle to push back while compressing the sphincter muscles at the same time. Patients with USI (loss of urine when straining, e.g., when coughing, sneezing, descending stairs) may lose urine involuntarily. When the patient's condition improves, there is no further loss of urine with this exercise.

Patients can use a shallow bowl (e.g., the Stabilizer from Sissel) to prevent the Swiss ball from rolling away. This makes the exercises safer for inexperienced and elderly patients. Bouncing and rocking movements are still possible with the ball in the bowl even when losing contact with the ball because it does not roll away.

14.6.6 Observation of Movements During Pelvic Floor Exercises

Movement Between Body and Ball. The primary impulse of a movement to perform an exercise is called the actio: the forward, backward, sideways, or diagonal rolling movement begins between the spherical form of the ischial tuberosities and the spherical form of the ball.

Because muscles of the pelvic and urogenital diaphragms arise from the bony parts of the pelvic floor, "gripping" the ball with the ischial tuberosities and pulling it forward (or backward, sideways, diagonally) can activate the muscles of the second and third layer as an actio.

Movement Within the Body. The movement continues into the hip joints and the lumbar spine, resulting in an extension of the hip joints and lumbar flexion with the forward rolling of the ball (flexion of the hips and extension of the lumbar spine with the backward rolling of the ball, lateral flexion trunk, and rotation of the pelvis over the thigh with sideways rolling).

To increase the intensity of the muscle activity it is important that the feet, knees, and thorax do not move. This confines the muscular activity to the pelvic floor, lower abdominal muscles, and low back.

Continuation of the Movement. The movement of the ischial tuberosities with the ball continues at the same time to change the contact area of the ball with the floor, resulting in the ball rolling forward, backward, sideways, or diagonally.

Limitation of the Movement. The extent of the total movement is limited by the thoracic spine, which remains in a neutral position, while the knees and the feet are spatially fixed.

> Neither the thorax nor the knees move in space, and the feet remain firmly planted on the floor. The movements can take place in a sagittal or frontal plane or a diagonal direction.

14.6.7 Final Observation and Practical Results

Patients generally wish to own their own Swiss ball in order to perform the exercises at home once the exercises have been learned under the supervision of a physical therapist. Regular follow-up visits in the physical therapy practice are necessary to adapt, change, and monitor the exercises and the patient's progress.

> For the patient it is very motivating to rediscover his own ability to move and enjoy movements which had been lost out of fear of incontinence.

The playful element of Swiss ball exercising, with its diversity of possibilities, allows goal-directed exercises while sitting on the ball during everyday situations. The patient obtains positive feedback. As a result the Swiss ball often becomes a trusted companion on the road to restoring the pelvic floor muscles. Many adults use the Swiss ball at home for their back problems already, and it is therefore easy to teach them its use for treating a "weak bladder."

Tanzberger's results over the past 10 years confirm that patients suffering pelvic floor insufficiencies and USI symptoms can achieve significant improvement within 3 months of beginning exercises, provided there is no neural damage, and the patient enjoys exercising.

> Once the patient has retrained the pelvic floor and the sphincter muscles there should be no need to continue exercising continuously unless he is unable to maintain the gains that have been achieved.

14.7 Description of Swiss Ball Exercises

While all exercises can be used with the various medical conditions described above, the therapist should individualize the exercises to the each patient's special needs and phases of recovery. The therapist may wish, for example, to work on increasing the resting tone of the levator ani and to strengthen the sphincter control of the urethra and the anus.

> Exercises such as "Roll-On" can help with the strengthening aspect, especially when pulling the ball in a forward direction (strengthening fibers which run in a sagittal direction). The backward rolling combined with inspiration may teach a person to relax tight muscle structures of the pelvic floor.
>
> Exercises such as "Kick and Kick" emphasize training of fast-twitch fibers, while exercises such as "Right Stop–Left Stop" activate muscle fibers of the pelvic floor that run in a frontal direction.
>
> Other exercises, such as "Draw a Urethra," train visual imaging and promote stability of the trunk while strengthening the pelvic floor muscles.

Eventually the patient should develop a good awareness of the pelvic floor and be able perform all the exercises, regardless of the nature of his original problem.

14.7.1 Exercises in the Sagittal Plane

Exercise examples:
- With the spine in a vertical position: variation with the Thera-Band (Fig. 14.10).
- With the stabilized spine leaning forward: "Lean Forward and Roll towards the Wall" (Fig. 14.8; or "Draw a Urethra," Fig. 14.9b).
- With the stabilized spine leaning backward: "Draw a Urethra" (Fig. 14.9a)

Starting Position. Sitting upright or leaning forward on the ball at approximately 90° hip and knee flexion. The legs are abducted at the hip joint and the feet keep contact with the floor.

Ball Size. Approximately 65 cm diameter, depending on the length of the patient's lower legs and his flexibility. The pressure must be firm.

Conditio. Instructions that help the patient to carry out the exercise are presented in Chap. 6. Flexion of the thoracic spine and dorsiflexion of the foot are limited if the knees are spatially fixed points and do not move, and the thoracic spine remains dynamically stabilized in extension.

Rhythm and Building of Tension. The pelvic floor and abdominal muscles support expiration. The ball and pelvic movement therefore changes with the rhythm of breathing.

Expiration

> The tension in the striated diaphragms and the sphincter muscles increases when the patient exhales against the resistance of stenosed lips for example, blowing "fffff," or when turning the tongue toward the roof of the palate and making a fricative sound such as "chchchch."

First Actio. The ball rolls forward during expiration.

First Reactio. The hip joints extend, the lumbar spine flexes, and the thoracic spine remains extended while the tension in the striated diaphragms and sphincter muscles increases.

Inspiration, Second Actio. During inspiration through the nose the ball rolls backward, the hip joints flex, the lumbar spine extends, and the thoracic spine remains extended (see also "Hula-Hula, Forward/Backward," Sect. 9.7).

Second Reactio. The pelvic floor relaxes.

Caution, Note

> At the end of the movement, which is limited by the conditios, the patient should maintain the position for approximately 1 second.

In exercises which provide continuous support with activation of the slow-twitch fibers the patient should hold the contraction 5–6 seconds, with a rest period of 10–15 seconds afterward (Wall et al. 1993).

> The patient is advised to visualize the tightening of the sphincter while exhaling and the letting go while inhaling.

Gestures with the hands describing the pelvic floor and sphincter movement may enhance the bodily awareness. The patient can also use a wand or Thera-Band while performing the exercises to stabilize the trunk at the same time.

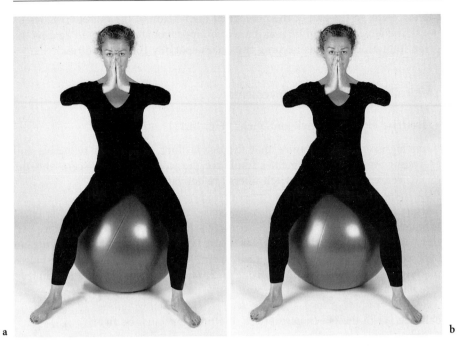

a   b

Fig. 14.6 a, b. "Right Stop–Left Stop." Starting and end position of exercise which trains pelvic floor and lateral trunk muscles. (Photographs by R. Tanzberger).

14.7.2 Exercises in the Frontal Plane

- Exercise example: "Right Stop–Left Stop" (Fig. 14.6).

Starting Position and Ball Pressure. As described in the previous exercise. To limit the lateral flexion of the trunk the patient lifts the arms in a transverse plane at the level of the shoulder girdle–chin, and presses the hands firmly together.

Ball Size. As described in previous exercise. The pressure must be firm.

Conditio. During the entire exercise the hands remain pressed firmly together. The spine remains in an upright posture (vertical), and the patient continues to breathe normally, emphasizing that there is no Valsalva maneuver.

Actio. One ischial tuberosity initiates the rolling movement to the opposite side, the right to the left side, then the left tuberosity to the right side (see also "Hula-Hula, Side to Side," Sect. 9.8).

Reactio. Tightening of the pelvic floor and sphincter muscles.

Caution, Note. At the end of the movement the tension of the muscle reaches its peak. The tension should be maintained for approximately 1 second against the given limitations such as keeping the knees spatially fixed (conditios).

14.7.3 Rocking/Bouncing Movements

- Exercise example: "Kick and Kick" (Fig. 14.11)

Bouncing exercises guarantee that the pelvic floor works in a reflective and ascending way. The movement stimuli are the weight of the viscera and the explosive expiration. Fast-twitch fibers are activated.

Starting Position. As in the previous exercise, the legs and feet are wide apart to increase the base of support. The lower legs and feet are in a vertical position. The spine is upright. The arms are in a transverse plane forming an oval at the level of the shoulder girdle–chin. To secure the position the ball is placed approximately 10 cm in front of a wall or in the Swiss ball stabilizer. The patient faces away from the wall.

Ball Size. As in the previous exercise, the pressure must be firm.

Actio. The feet press firmly into the floor, the pelvis bounces vertically up and away from the ball, and the arms move from sideways to foreward and upward. The patient pronounces the explosive word "kick" (during expiration) when the pelvis and the pelvic floor lose contact with the ball. During the second word, "and," the patient rocks the pelvis, bouncing twice in order to lift off again with the next "kick." The sound of this is: "kick aaaaand kick aaaaand kick aaaaand kick" etc.

Reactio. The pelvic floor is activated as a reaction to the stimulus of the bouncing movement, the explosive expiration, and the weight of the viscera.

Caution, Note. Until the patient feels more secure, this exercise can be practiced on the PhysioRoll. The arms can make hand gestures such as the closure of the urogenital hiatus to stimulate a visual image of closing of the muscles.

 The pelvis loses contact with the ball, so use caution!

The patient's safety is always most important. The knee joints change the angle of flexion by approximately 30° when bouncing, but extension should not be allowed. The "Cowboy" exercise (Sect. 9.1) can be used to train elements of this exercise.

From the above exercise models many further exercises can be devised. Other exercises, such as the "Easter Bunny" (Sect. 9.26) and "Well Figure" (9.27) can also be adapted for use in pelvic floor exercises.

14.8 Exercise Examples

The following exercise examples are performed in various planes.

14.8.1 "Roll-On"

This exercise is performed in a sagittal plane (Fig. 14.5).

Goals. Increase in muscle tonus in the urogenital diaphragm and urethral sphincter muscle.

Ball Size. The diameter of the ball must allow the patient to sit upright on the ball, with feet, knees, and hips at 90° (usually the ball size is at least 65 cm, but this depends on the length of the lower legs and mobility of the hip joints). The pressure must be firm to allow easy rolling.

Starting Position. The patient sits upright on the ball. The legs are wide apart, the feet press firmly into the ground, and the lower legs are spatially vertical. The lumbar spine is extended. The stable trunk leans forward (flexion in the hip joints), the hands are positioned on the thigh to support the weight of the trunk, and the elbows remain flexed throughout the exercise.

First Actio. The ischial tuberosities initiate the movement and roll the ball in a forward direction (ventrally); the lumbar spine flexes. At the same time the patient exhales, stenosing the glottis and producing a fricative sound such as "chchchch ..." (no vocal sounds).

First Reactio. Concentric activity of the lower abdominal muscles and pelvic floor activity, with increase in muscle tonus of the sagittal fibers in particular (e.g., of the pubococcygeus muscle).

Second Actio. The ischial tuberosities roll the ball in a straight line backward; the knees do not move (they are spatially fixed points). The patient inhales through the nose.

Second Reactio. Concentric extension of the lumbar spine while maintaining muscle tonus of the pelvic floor.

Caution, Note

| | The exercise is especially helpful with men after prostatectomy. |

14.8.2 "Right Stop–Left Stop"

This exercise is performed in a frontal plane (Fig. 14.6).

Goals. Improved muscle tonus of pelvic floor and lateral trunk muscles.

Ball Size. As described in previous exercises.

Starting Position. The patient sits upright on the ball, as described in the previous exercises. The legs are approximately hip-width apart, the lower legs spatially vertical, the feet firmly planted on the floor. The palm of the hands are pressed together in front of the chin, with the arms in a transverse plane at the level of the shoulders.

Actio. The initial movement comes from the ischial tuberosities, which roll the ball to the right or the left side in a frontal plane. The knees remain spatially fixed points. When reaching the "stop" position on the right or left side, the patient says "stooop" to intensify the muscle activity. The patient also visualizes the ball to be very heavy and the tuberosity of each side must make a great effort to move it.

Reactio. Increased tension of the pelvic floor and lateral trunk muscles (e.g., quadratus lumborum, transverse abdominus, oblique abdominus muscles).

Caution, Note. See also the exercise "Hula-Hula, Side to Side" (Sect. 9.8), which can be practiced as preparation for this exercise.

14.8.3 "Sit Upright and Roll Toward the Wall"

The exercise is performed in the sagittal plane (Fig. 14.7).

Goals. Training of the sphincter muscles. Concentric training of sagittal fibers of the pelvic floor and strengthening of the lower abdominal muscles.

Ball Size. As described in the exercise "Roll-On."

Starting Position. The patient sits off-center on the anterior part of the ball and faces a straight wall. The ball is approximately 15 cm away from the wall, and the inside of the feet and the knees touch the wall. The hands are placed on the thigh in close proximity of the hip joints; the elbows are flexed and pointing backward. The thoracic spine is extended.

Actio. The ischial tuberosities initiate the movement and roll the ball toward the wall. At the same time the patient exhales with a long "chchchch ... ."

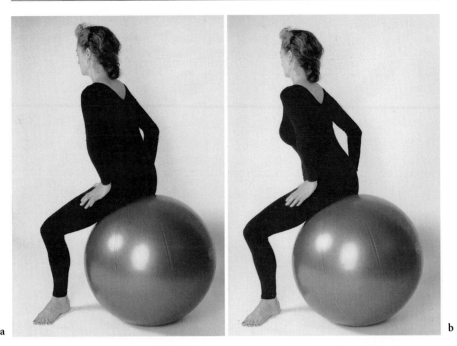

a   b

Fig. 14.7 a, b. "Sit Upright and Roll Toward the Wall." Starting and end position. The exercise trains predominantly the sphincter muscles. (Photographs by R. Tanzberger).

The patient also visualizes, first, the anal muscles all tightening as a cuff, then the vaginal muscles, and finally the urethral muscles.

Reactio. Flexion of the lumbar spine and some extension of the pelvis in the hip joints. Concentric strengthening (by tightening) of the sphincter muscles of anus, vagina, and urethra.

Return Actio. When returning to the starting position, the knees remain in contact with the wall while the ischial tuberosities move the ball in a straight line backward.

Return Reactio. Concentric activity of the back extensor muscles, relaxation of the pelvic floor muscles.

Caution, Note. The contact of the knees with the wall during the forward and the backward movements must remain constant and firm.

14.8.4 "Lean Forward and Roll Toward the Wall"

This exercise is performed in the sagittal plane (Fig. 14.8).

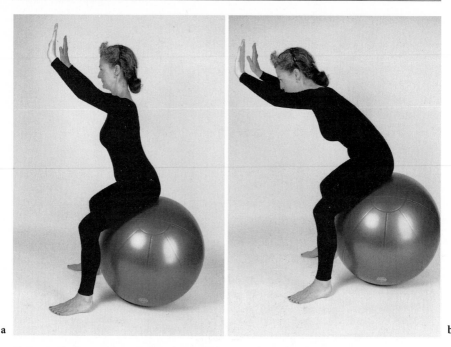

a
b

Fig. 14.8 a, b. "Lean forward and Roll Toward the Wall" starting and end position. The exercise strengthens sphincter muscles. (Photographs by R. Tanzberger).

Goals. Training of the sphincter muscles. Concentric training of sagittal fibers of the pelvic floor and strengthening of the lower abdominal muscles.

Ball Size. As described in the exercise "Roll-On."

Starting Position. The patient sits off-center on the anterior part of the ball and faces the wall. The ball is approximately 40 cm away from the wall, with the legs spread apart. The trunk leans forward, and the hands are supported on the wall approximately at the level of the head. The elbows are slightly flexed. The distance of the knees to the wall remains constant throughout the exercise.

Actio. The ischial tuberosities initiate the movement and roll the Swiss ball toward the wall. At the same time the patient exhales with a long "chchchch …" and visualizes voluntarily tightening the urethral muscles as a cuff, then the vaginal muscles tightening and closing as a cuff, and finally the dynamic tightening of the anal muscles.

> The patient should have an "inner picture" of these activities.

During the actio the dynamic stability of the thoracic spine does not change (conditio: the distance between navel and sternal notch remains the same).

Reactio. Contraction of the sphincter muscles.

Return Actio. When the patient rolls backward to the starting position, he inhales.

Return Reactio. Relaxation of muscle tension. The lumbar spine extends and the thoracic spine maintains its dynamic stability.

Caution, Note. The knees remain spatial fixed points and do not move.

14.8.5 "Draw a Urethra"

This exercise is performed in a sagittal plane (Fig. 14.9).

Goals. Training of the sphincter muscles through visualization. Reactive abdominal and pelvic floor muscle strengthening by changing rhythmically from tension to relaxation.

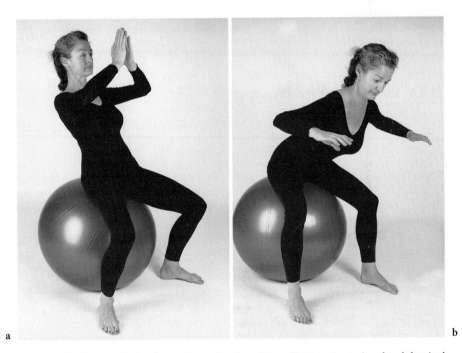

a   b

Fig. 14.9a,b. "Draw a Urethra." Starting and end position. The exercise trains the abdominal and pelvic floor muscles reactively. (Photographs by R. Tanzberger).

Ball Size. As described in the exercise "Roll-On."

Starting Position. The patient sits upright on the ball, as described in previous exercises. The legs are wide apart, the feet press firmly into the ground, and the lower legs are spatially vertical. The lumbar spine is extended.

First Actio. The dynamically stable trunk leans backward while the Swiss ball rolls forward. The patient visualizis a narrow and erekt urethra, while the hands draw the picture of a urethra in the air. The patient exhales with the fricative sound "chchchch … ."

Conditio. No increase in pressure under the feet.

First Reactio. Increased tension of the pelvic floor and abdominal muscles.

Second Actio. With inhalation through the nose the dynamically stable spine leans forward, while the ball rolls backward. The arms and hands open and move to the side in a transverse plane at the level of the shoulders.

Second Reactio. Relaxation of the pelvic floor muscles while stabilizing the back extensor muscles.

Caution, Note. The exercise "Scale" (Sect. 9.2) can be used to prepare the patient for this exercise.

14.8.6 Variation with the Thera-Band

This exercise is performed with minimal movement in a sagittal plane (Fig. 14.10).

Goals. Training of the sphincter muscles through visualization. Strengthening of abdominal, back extensor, and pelvic floor muscles reactively by changing rhythmically from tension to relaxation while leaning the trunk backward and forward. Stabilization of the trunk.

Ball Size. As described in the exercise "Roll-On."

Starting Position. The patient sits upright on the center of the ball, as described in previous exercises. The legs are hip-width apart and the feet press firmly into the Thera-Band placed under the feet. The arms are above the head, pulling the Thera-Band toward the ceiling and backward. The lumbar spine is extended; the thoracic spine is dynamically stable in neutral. The lower legs are vertical; the knees spatially fixed points.

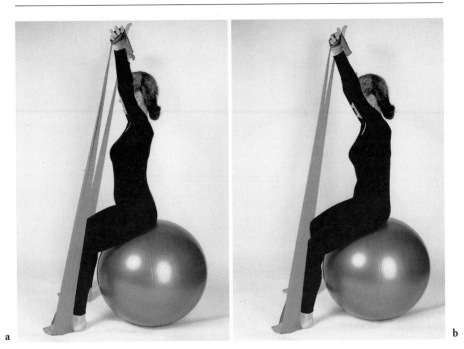

a   b

Fig. 14.10 a, b. "Variation with the Thera-Band." Starting and end position. The exercise strengthens pelvic floor muscles while maintaining trunk stability. (Photographs by R. Tanzberger).

Actio. The ischial tuberosities pull the ball in a forward direction toward the heels while maintaining the neutral position of the thoracic spine. The lumbar spine flexes.

Reactio. The lower abdominal muscles are activated concentrically. The pelvic floor muscles and the sphincter muscles tighten and support the movement.

Caution, Note. As described in the previous exercises, the movement can be combined with breathing and visualization. The tension of the Thera-Band varies depending on the strength of the patient. The patient can also use two Thera-Bands under each foot. The Thera-Band can be stretched diagonally or horizontally at shoulder level in an imaginary frontal plane which passes through the knees.

14.8.7 "Kick and Kick"

This exercise moves the patient in a vertical direction (Fig. 14.11).

Goals. Reactive tightening and relaxation of the pelvic floor and sphincter muscles while bouncing up and down. Activation of fast-twitch fibers of the levator ani muscle.

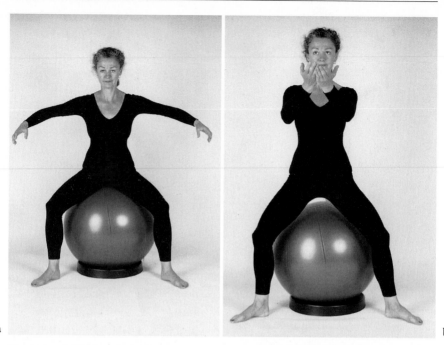

Fig. 14.11 a,b. "Kick and Kick." Starting and end position. The exercise strengthens the pelvic floor and sphincter muscles while bouncing up and down. (Photographs by R. Tanzberger).

Ball Size. As described in the exercise "Roll-On."

Starting Position. The patient sits upright on the ball, which is placed in a Sissel Stabilizer to prevent it from rolling away. The patient's arms are abducted and elevated at shoulder level. The legs are abducted; the lower legs are spatially vertical (the knees spatially fixed points). The feet press firmly against the floor.

Actio. When the patient begins to bounce by pushing off from the feet, the hands move into a midsagittal plane and simulate a lifting movement. The patient then visualizes the pelvic floor tightening and lifting. The upward bouncing is accompanied with the explosive word "kick"; when coming down again, the patient says "and." Then once more "kick" when bouncing up again.

Reactio. The pelvic floor and sphincter muscles tighten reactively, holding the weight of the viscera. There is also a bridge activity of the pelvic floor sphincter muscles (see Fig. 14.11b). As a reaction to the explosive "kick" pressure is exerted on the pelvic floor, and reactive tightening of the muscles is thus stimulated.

Caution, Note. It is important to prevent the ball from rolling away. The exercise can be performed in a corner, with the therapist providing safety by placing a rolled blanket or towel around the base of the ball or by having a person stand by. The patient can vary the intensity of the bouncing. The exercise can be used as a test for continence and also to demonstrate improvement from incontinence. The "Cowboy" exercise (see Sect. 9.1) prepares the patient for "Kick and Kick."

Therapists can develop their own variations on the basis of these exercises that are adapted to the individual patient's needs.

References

Adams C, Frahm J (1995) Genitourinary System. In: Myers RS (ed) Manual of physical therapy practice. Saunders, Philadelphia, pp 459–504

Basmajian JV, De Luca CJ (1985) Anterior abdominal wall and peritoneum. In: Muscles alive. Williams & Wilkins, Baltimore, pp 389–407

Bø K, Hagen RH, Kvarstein B, Jørgensen J, Larsen S (1990) Pelvic floor muscle exercise for the treatment of female stress urinary incontinence. III. Effects of two different degrees of pelvic floor muscle exercises. Neurourol Urodynam 9:489

Bump RC, Hurt GW, Fantl A, Wyman JF (1991) Assessment of Kegel pelvic muscle exercise performance after brief verbal instruction. Am J Obstet Gynecol 165:322–329

Byl NN, Merzenich MM, Cheung S, Bedenbaugh P, Nagarajan SS, Jenkins WM (1997) A primate model for studying focal dystonia and repetitive strain injury: effects on the the primary somatosensory cortex. Physical Ther 77(3):269–284

Cunningham FG, MacDonald PC, Leveno KJ, Gant NF, Gilstrap III LC (1993) Anatomy of the reproductive tract in women. In: Williams' obstetrics, 19th edn. Appleton & Lange, Norwalk, pp 57–79

Elia G, Bergman A (1993) Pelvic muscle exercises: when do they work? Obstet Gynecol 81:283–286

Henalla SM, Kirwan P, Castleden CM, Hutchins CJ, Breeson AJ (1988) The effect of pelvic floor exercises in the treatment of genuine urinary stress incontinence in women at two hospitals. Br J Obstet Gynaecol 95:602–606

Holley RL, Varner ER, Kerns DJ, Mestecky PJ (1995) Long-term failure of pelvic floor musculature exercises in treatment of genuine stress incontinence. South Med J 88(5):547–549

Jäning W (1995) Vegetatives Nervensystem. In: Schmidt RF, Thews G (eds) Physiologie des Menschen, 26th edn. Springer, Berlin Heidelberg New York, pp 357–363

Kegel AH (1948) Progressive resistance exercises in the functional restoration of the perineal muscles. Am J Obstet Gynecol 8:238–348

Kegel AH (1951) Physiologic therapy for urinary stress incontinence. JAMA 163(10):915–917

Kegel AH, Powell TO (1950) The physiological treatment of urinary stress incontinence. J Urolog 63(5):808–813

Klein-Vogelbach S (1990) Functional kinetics. Springer, Berlin Heidelberg New York

Klein-Vogelbach S (1991) Therapeutic exercises in functional kinetics. Springer, Berlin Heidelberg New York

Krüger H-J, Krüger G (1991) Harninkontinenz – eine soziokulturelle Erkrankung? Krankengymnastik 43(12):1345–1348

McCandless S, Mason G (1995) Physical therapy as an effective change agent in the treatment of patients with urinary incontinence. J Mississippi Med Assoc 9:271–274

McIntosh LJ, Frahm JD, Mallett VT, Richardson DA (1993) Pelvic floor rehabilitation in the treatment of incontinence. J Repr Med 38(9):662–665

the thoracic spine become reactively hypotonic, while the upper abdominal and probably scalene muscles (which must then hold the weight of the thorax) become reactively hypertonic. The upper part of the trapezius muscles become reactively hypertonic because they must hold the weight of the forward head.

Postural alignment, good strength and mobility of the trunk and extremities are essential to standing, walking erect, and using the arms and legs without causing unnecessary strain. The dynamic stability of the trunk when leaning forward or backward is of paramount importance to protect the spine from undue strain whether in sitting or standing, and whether quietly vertical or during dynamic weight shifting. In their development and function, movements of the body affect the human being as a whole, and posture and orofacial movements affect the shaping of the jaw and the formation of sounds (Broich 1996). This can be imagined when observing the posture of the boy in Fig. 11.18, whose treatment certainly could be considered as much preventative as rehabilitative.

The Alexander technique (Blum 1995; Rosenthal 1987) was developed by an Australian actor and singer in the early part of this century when he recognized how his posture and lack of body awareness affected his voice. The Alexander technique emphasizes the restoration of correct posture through unconscious and conscious learning. Similar observations have also been made by Feldenkrais (Nelson 1989) and Klein-Vogelbach (1990, 1991).

> Faulty movement patterns become subconscious and automatic but lack efficiency and may cause pain. These habits can be altered by gaining awareness of them.

> Many persons choose their profession without knowing whether they are physically able to perform the job, and whether their strength and mobility is sufficient to carry out the work that it entails.

A violinist, for example, should have back muscles that are strong enough to maintain the stability of the trunk while standing and leaning forward with both arms elevated in front of the body. The weight of the instrument adds to the weight of the arms which must be lifted while playing. Without strong trunk muscles, the muscles of the shoulder girdle may try to compensate, and if there is also faulty alignment of pelvis, thorax, and head, pain is the inevitable result.

A nurse or physical therapist working in acute care must have excellent general strength, apply good body mechanics, and be very skillful in lifting, turning, pulling, and transferring heavy patients. The incidence of back pain resulting in musculoskeletal disorders is high in these professions (Bork et al. 1996). Nurses and physical therapists are not tested during their schooling for their physical fitness to fulfill these job requirements, and unless they acquire good mobility, strength, and skill and use proper body mechanics, the chances are high that they will injure their backs during the course of their job.

Back and neck pain is also common in other occupations, such as those of bus drivers and factory workers, and its prevalence is so great that it constitutes a major health problem in both industrial and preindustrial societies (Anderson 1992).

Working out in the gymnasium is very popular with many adults. Unfortunately, increasing muscle strength is often their main focus.

> Healthy persons do not realize how their lack of mobility can affect them adversely during strength training, especially when working out in poor posture. Faulty movement patterns are often reinforced, and frequently these exercises lack mobility and skill and may lead to injuries.

Faulty mobility can be a major factor in producing pain. For example, hypomobility restricts movement in one segment of the spine and causes greater movement in another segment.

> The pain often occurs in the hypermobile segment. Because movement is a physiological system, dysfunctions in this system must be alleviated or faulty movement can otherwise induce pathology (Sahrman 1993).

Muscle spasms can cause strain to fascias and joints and may affect joint position, cause strain to the soft tissue, and impair the central nervous motor programming (Janda 1991). This excessive stress to all structures of the musculoskeletal system is a precondition for the development of chronic pain syndromes.

> The conclusions that can be drawn from this discussion are:
> - For healthy adults who want to prevent injuries to the musculoskeletal system, it is of paramount importance to maintain normal mobility of the joints, soft tissue, and neural structures to be able to move and exercise in proper alignment.
> - Good posture during sitting, standing, and movement can help prevent injuries to the musculoskeletal system.
> - Extremities and trunk muscles should be strengthened in proper alignment only (not in faulty movement patterns).
> - It is important to strengthen not only the superficial muscles of the trunk but also the intrinsic muscles, which act as stabilizers and help prevent overuse of muscles attached to the shoulder girdle.

15.2 Evaluating Postural Alignment in Healthy Persons

Standard posture is consistent with sound scientific principles, involves minimal amount of stress and strain, and is conducive to maximal efficiency of the body. From the posterior view of a standing person a plumb line coincides with the spinous processes and the midsagittal plane of the head. In side view the plumb line ends slightly in front of the lateral malleolus and also passes through most of the bodies of the cervical and lumbar vertebrae and the shoulder joint and slightly posterior to the frontotransverse axis of the hip joint (Kendall et al. 1993).

Many factors affect posture, and these must all be considered when evaluating a patient, including his proportions (length, width, depth, and weight of body segments), constitution, and acquired weight (e.g., obesity; Klein-Vogelbach 1990). Therapists must also assess hyper- and hypomobility of joints as this contributes to the development of dysfunctions of the musculoskeletal system. The therapist is thus able to identify movement restrictions that may lead to problems. Suggestions for evaluation and treatment that enable the therapist to recognize movement and strength deficits are provided by Kendall et al. (1993), Klein-Vogelbach (1990), and Janda (1994). Examining a patient's typical posture at work may supply the therapist with additional information about movement and strength deficits.

Breathing Pattern

> In normal breathing the abdomen expands with inspiration around the waist line. The movement then extends to the lower ribs, which widen with inspiration and narrow with expiration.

In faulty breathing patterns the chest raises first, which increases the tension and strain to the neck muscles, in particular the scalene muscles. This faulty breathing pattern is frequently associated with neck pain and thoracic outlet syndrome.

After evaluating posture and movement the therapist decides whether the patient is in need of stretching/mobilization or strengthening/stabilization and chooses exercises which address the postural deficits that have been identified.

> Although some persons are sufficiently aware of posture and movement to correct such deficits without assistance, most do indeed require a therapist's help.

The following elements of good posture can be pointed out to the person.

Distribution of Body Weight

Body weight should be evenly distributed over the feet, neither more on the heels nor on the forefeet, and neither on the one leg nor on the other. The person must first feel how the weight can be shifted to the heels or the toes or from one foot to the other. The person's hands can be used to feel that the body distances of the trunk do not change while shifting the weight over the feet (see Sect. 5.6). Until the patient becomes independent, he can self-correct under the supervision and with cues from a therapist. In order to match cognition with cerebellar synergy programming, which most likely leads to quicker learning, the person should also try to *close the eyes and feel* his body.

Base of Support

In ideal posture the heels are approximately 3 in. (7–8 cm) apart (Kendall 1993). A narrower base of support normally increases the strain to the back; a wider base may be useful when performing a job in standing (e.g., vacuum cleaning). In standing the change of muscle tonus can be palpated in the small of the back for the back extensor muscles or near the sternal notch for the neck flexor muscles. When standing on the toes, especially when swaying slightly, the muscles feel tighter than when the feet are apart and planted firmly on the floor.

Muscle Length and Weakness

Tightness of hamstring muscles can be recognized in supine position. A person should be able to raise one leg straight to approximately 80°. Tightness of the hip flexor muscles is likely when a person has a very pronounced lordosis in standing. If the lordosis increases when kneeling, the shortness is principally in the rectus femoris muscles. It is important that the person understands and feels *the faulty and correct postures* in order to appreciate the difference.

> Increased lordosis is frequently associated with overstretched and weak abdominal muscles and tight back muscles.

Since most persons like having strong abdominal muscles, they are usually very willing to learn proper exercising.

> **EXAMPLES**
>
> Stretching the hip-flexor muscles correctly should be felt in the anterior aspect of the thigh, never in the low back. If, while stretching the rectus femoris muscle, the heel is pulled toward the buttocks, the person may perform an evasive movement, by tilting the pelvis ante-

> riorly, which results in an increased lordosis of the low back and pos-
> sible pain there. If performed correctly, there is a posterior or no tilt
> of the pelvis.
> A better instruction is to move the buttock away from the heel (or
> the *hip joint* in a forward direction), which may also activate the low-
> er abdominal muscles. This most likely can be felt as a stretch of the
> rectus femoris in the anterior aspect of the thigh. A healthy person
> may first want to try the correct and incorrect ways to increase his
> awareness and ability to self-correct.

Healthy persons with forward shoulders usually have shortness of the pectorales muscles, which results in weakness of the middle part of the trapezius
muscle. By learning to move the shoulders many times throughout the day
into the midfrontal plane of the body the person can strengthen the middle
part of the trapezius muscle and improve his posture. Stretching of the pectoral muscles can be performed as well.

> A forward head is often associated with tightness of the upper trape-
> zius muscles, forward shoulders, and a trunk which appears to lean
> backward. Again, it may be helpful to let the patient palpate the dif-
> ference in muscle tonus in the neck or back, in both poor and cor-
> rected postures to increase his awareness.

Growing numbers of personal trainers use the Swiss ball for their clients. Vi-
deotapes are available for healthy persons demonstrating the use of the Swiss
ball for low-impact aerobics, stretching, and strengthening exercises (Posner-
Mayer and Zappala 1993).

The Swiss ball therefore contributes to an enjoyable work-out and is a valuable tool for home use in both preventative and corrective therapeutic in-
terventions.

15.3 Applications to Prevent Injury of the Musculoskeletal System

Treatment Plan

- To stretch and mobilize tight structures of soft tissue, neural tissue and
  joints
- To strengthen muscles in a functional reactive way so good movement
  patterns become automatic
- To increase proprioceptive awareness of good postural alignment
- To train balance, coordination, and skill

After evaluating standing, sitting, and work positions, the therapist can use
the Swiss ball.

Treatment Goals

- To achieve normal mobility of tight structures (soft tissue, neural tissue, muscles, and joints)
- To obtain normal muscle strength, especially of muscles that must perform antigravity stabilization in work-related positions
- To train proprioceptive awareness in good alignment while sitting or standing
- To achieve good balance, coordination, and skill to enable a healthy person to react quickly without straining the body

15.4 Treatment Examples

 Caution: Care must be taken with weight-bearing exercises on the hands if there are symptoms at the forearms, wrists, or hands.

15.4.1 A Dental Hygienist

A slightly overweight female dental hygienist often leaned and turned to the left side when working. She complained of aches and pains in the back and neck at the end of the day but had received no treatment. Her strength appeared to be within normal limits.

It is not surprising that many dentists and dental hygienists complain of aches and pains of the back and neck as they must frequently work in a position which requires an asymmetrical posture. If such persons can restore and maintain flexibility and symmetry of the posture, they can probably prevent fixed postural deviations and reduce aches and pains.

EXAMPLES

Figure 15.1. A dental hygienist demonstrates her typical working posture. She bends to the side, rotates to the left, and lacks spinal extension. The flexed posture may also compromise expansion of the lungs and lead to fatigue. At times this flexed posture irritates the stomach.
Figure 15.2. Panel a. Side bending of the trunk and neck while sitting shows good mobility to the left side (working posture).
Panel b. Side bending of the trunk and neck to the right side is limited and can be measured by the greater distance from the right elbow to the floor than from the left elbow to the floor (compare panel a). Side bending of the neck is reduced as well.
In both panels the upper arm is almost vertical in space; while the head in is tilted almost horizontally in panel a, it is tilted only approximately 45° in panel b.

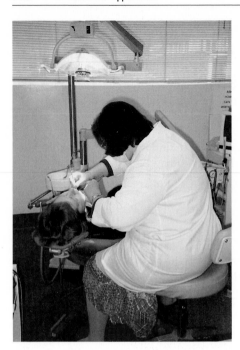

Fig. 15.1. A dental hygienist demonstrates her typical working posture. She is side-bent and rotated to the left side and lacks spinal extension.

> *Figure 15.3.* Panel a. When the patient bends to the left, a harmonious arc can be observed, with the arm reaching over the head while the trunk elongates.
>
> Panel b. Lateral flexion to the right side is considerably limited, probably due to tightness of soft tissue and muscles and resulting in tightness of neural structures.
>
> The rightward side-bending position in this person is good for mobilizing tight soft tissue and muscles of the left side of the trunk.

Such differences in movement ability between the two sides of the body can contribute to aches and pains at the end of the working day and may even lead to chronic pain if movement is not restored. Physical therapists must be alert to the danger from repetitive strain and overuse. Low back pain may be due, for example, to tightness of the quadratus lumborum and the latissimus muscles. There is also potential for neck pain and neural problems in the right arm if mobility is not restored.

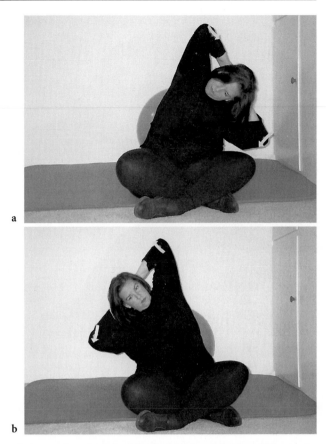

Fig. 15.2 a. Side bending of the trunk and neck while sitting shows good mobility to the left side (working posture). **b.** Side bending of the trunk and neck to the right side is limited and can be measured by the increased distance of the right elbow to the floor compared to the left elbow to the floor in the previous figure.

Figure 15.4. Panel a. The Swiss ball (65 cm diameter) is used to mobilize the spine into rotation to the right side while strengthening abdominal muscles.

Panel b. The hips are spatially fixed points while the trunk is extended, the left arm is pushing the ball forward, and there is an element of rotation if the patient looks under her left arm. The right hand is placed at shoulder level on the floor.

Panel c. With both arms and the forehead resting on the ball, extension of the spine is practiced with the assistance of gravity as the hips remain spatially fixed points.

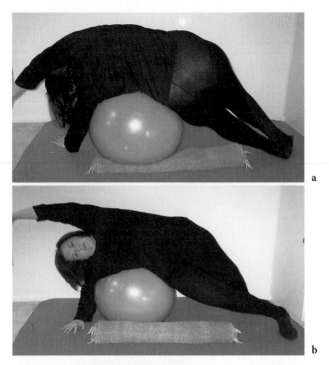

Fig. 15.3. a While side bending to the left side, a harmonious arc can be observed, the arm reaches over the head of the elongated trunk. **b.** Lateral flexion to the right side is considerably limited, probably due to tightness of soft tissue and muscles and resulting in tightness of neural structures.

The dental hygienist would also benefit from strengthening her intrinsic back muscles (see Chapters 11, 12). Many exercises described in Chapter 9 can be adapted to benefit this person [e.g., the "Salamander" (Sect. 9.9), "Scissors" (9.19), "Carrousel" (9.21), "Mermaid" (9.20), "Cowboy" (9.1), "Goldfish" (9.15), "Donkey Stretch Yourself" (9.4)] as these exercises increase mobility of the spine and strengthen the trunk muscles, while also providing proprioceptive input for a good posture.

15.4.2 Musicians

Musicians frequently suffer from musculoskeletal and neuromuscular conditions (Bejjani et al. 1996). Thoracic outlet syndrome is a relatively common cause of upper extremity symptoms among instrumental musicians (Lederman 1987). Orchestral musicians are usually committed to playing up to 30 hours per week in rehearsals and concerts, each lasting up to 3 hours, and many simply accept the accompanying pain as a normal condition.

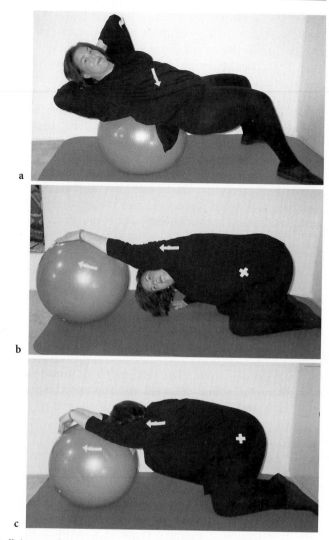

Fig. 15.4 a. The Swiss ball (65 cm diameter) is used to mobilize the spine into rotation to the right side while strengthening abdominal muscles. **b.** The hips are spatially fixed points while the trunk is extended; the left arm is pushing the ball forward. **c.** With both arms and the forehead resting on the ball, extension of the spine is practiced.

Overuse syndromes are found in over 50% of orchestral players (Fry 1986). However, most neuromusculoskeletal problems of instrumental musicians are preventable or amenable to minor modifications in technique or environment (Sandin 1989).

In cases of acute inflammatory or overuse injury the key to treatment is rest for at least 2–3 days. In addition to nonsteroid anti-inflammatory agents, "A knowledgeable therapist can be very helpful in assisting patients with carry-over of exercise, pointing out postural problems of which the patient may not be aware, motivating the patient, and structuring the patient's progress" (Sandin 1989).

The problems encountered specifically by musicians are dealt with by Byl and Arriaga (1993), who discuss evaluation, treatment, adapting playing technique for various instruments, as well as the role of inadequate seating, eating, and sleeping habits. Too little attention is given to problems that are aggravated by poor seating; concert musicians seldom have a choice in se-lecting a chair that would be adequate to their size and proportions. When standing, they often place their feet too close together and thereby establish a base of support for themselves that is too small.

> However, many musicians with back pain cannot maintain a good posture over a period of time because they lack flexibility and strength of their musculoskeletal system.

Flexibility, strength, balance and coordination can be practiced preventatively with the Swiss ball.

> Observing a musician performing or practicing music can help the therapist to find areas which, if ignored, can cause the patient prob-lems and functional disabilities if allowed to persist for long periods of time.

> **Caution:** Special care must be taken to avoid stressing the hands and wrists; exercises that emphasize weight-bearing on hands should therefore be avoided. Exercises should not cause pain.

The first treatment example (Figs. 15.5, 15.6) is that of a female violinist, who complained that "my shoulder/neck is killing me." Whenever the violin-ist rehearsed and played frequently in concerts, she complained of this nag-ging pain. Using the Swiss ball helped the violinist to alleviate pain during and after practice and rehearsals.

EXAMPLES

Figure 15.5. The violinist demonstrates her posture while practicing for a concert. Both arms are elevated, and their weight and the weight of the instrument must be stabilized primarily by the back muscles. The head is in a slight forward position, both shoulders elevated. The violinist has a good base of support and her hip flexion is at least 90°, which is adequate.

Fig. 15.5. The violinist demonstrates her posture while practicing for a concert. Both arms are elevated and their weight and the weight of the instrument must be stabilized primarily by the back muscles.

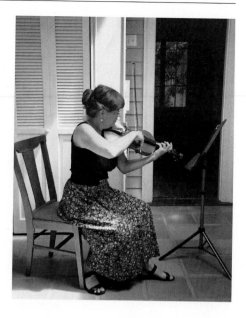

Musicians who lack good active hip flexion (normal is 120°–130°) may benefit from sitting on a wedge, which allows more flexion at the hip joints when leaning forward.

The recommendation for this violinist was to take frequent breaks when practicing and to perform preventative exercises with the Swiss ball and foam roll after the practice session to stabilize the trunk in neutral, mobilize it in extension (with a pillow under the head to avoid hyperextension of the neck), and create body awareness for symmetry. Other parts of the exercises were gently stretching the pectoral muscles and proprioceptive training for good postural alignment.

Below are some exercises which helped the violinist:

EXAMPLES

Figure 15.6. Panel a. Lying supine over a Swiss ball (65 cm diameter), the patient stretches her pectoral muscles, mobilizes her spine into extension, and balances the trunk. She chooses a wide base of support; her legs are placed apart. To increase balance and symmetry (as a progression) the violinist can move her legs closer together.

Panel b. Lying supine on a foam roll with the feet placed on the ball, the arms abducted in approximately 90°, the patient creates awareness for symmetry. She also stretches her pectoral muscles, and by pressing her hands and heels against an imaginary wall (adapted from the Brunkow concept, Bold and Grossman 1989) she achieves cocontraction of muscles in trunk and extremities.

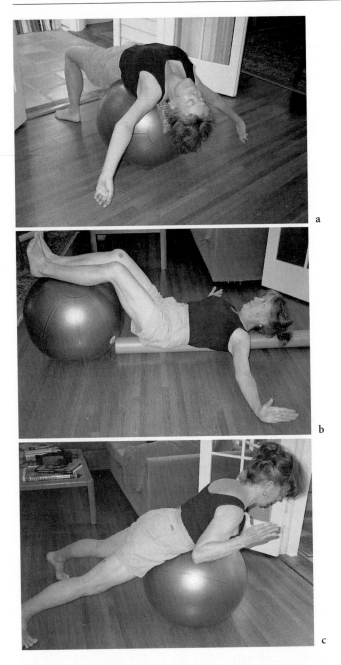

Fig. 15.6 a. Lying supine over a Swiss ball (65 cm diameter) the patient stretches her pectoral muscles, mobilizes her spine into extension, and balances the trunk. **b.** Lying supine on a foam roll with the feet placed on the ball, the arms abducted in approximately 90°. **c.** Prone over the Swiss ball, the musician works on strengthening and stabilizing the trunk extensor muscles against gravity.

> Panel c. Prone over the Swiss ball, the musician strengthens and sta-
> bilizes the trunk extensor muscles against gravity. Balance, postural
> alignment, symmetry, and shoulder depression are trained with this
> exercise, which is adapted from the "Figurehead" (Sect. 9.18). The
> feet are placed wide apart to increase the base of support. As a pro-
> gression, the base of support can be decreased.

The second example for the treatment of musicians presents a female pianist
(Fig. 15.7).

EXAMPLES

> *Figure 15.7.* The woman learns postural alignment while sitting on an
> unstable base of support (a Swiss ball). This helps her to improve an
> awareness for good posture while playing. As a progression, bouncing
> in good alignment may be added and the feet can be placed closer to-
> gether.
> The pianist was also instructed to "pretend" playing piano while sit-
> ting on the Swiss ball. The pianist then needed to move from the
> compliant surface of the ball to the hard surface of the piano bench
> and actually practice playing the piano in order to guarantee func-
> tional carryover to a task-specific activity.

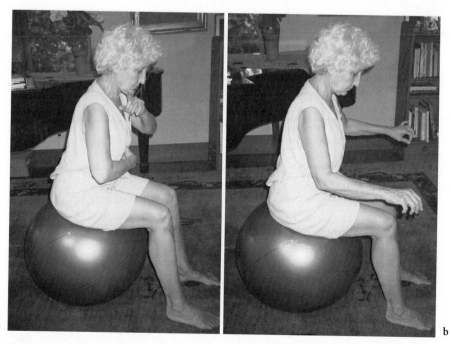

a   b

Fig. 15.7. A female pianist learns postural alignment while sitting on an unstable base of
support before practicing piano sitting on a hard surface.

There are many more exercises that musicians can perform to train balance, strength, and proprioception. Before playing music, bouncing upright on the ball can provide proprioceptive input for postural alignment, and leaning the stable trunk forward and back trains dynamic stability of the spine [e.g., "Cowboy" (Sect. 9.1) and "Scale" (Sect. 9.2)].

15.4.3 Desk/Computer Workers

There are many other professions in which Swiss ball exercises can help persons overcome aches and pains during or after a stressful day at work. Seated work can in fact cause as much pain and dysfunction as lifting (Lear and Pomeroy 1994). The following example is of a person who sat most of the day at a desk in front of a computer.

EXAMPLES

Figure 15.8. Panel a. A young writer who works out in a gymnasium several times a week to strengthen his muscles spent most of his working day at the computer. His sitting posture demonstrated poor postural alignment and insufficient mobility, and that may cause aches and pain.

Tilting the chair backward results in a compensatory forward head posture. Neck and back pain are a possible consequence unless mobility (especially of the hip joints into flexion, the upper trunk into extension) and postural alignment are improved.

Instead of moving the pelvis forward and dynamically stabilizing the trunk, the head is pulled forward. The writer probably has short hamstring and neck extensor muscles and diminished dynamic stability of the trunk and mobility of the spine in extension and rotation (a flexed spine does not rotate easily). The young man did not feel or see that he had the potential for developing back pain, because his body awareness is decreased.

Panel b. The writer demonstrates that even in a small office the Swiss ball can be used to mobilize the spine into extension by placing the ball on top of the desk.

Panel c. Rolling the Swiss ball backward while leaning with the forearms on the desk helps to extend the back while flexing the hips. Lack of good flexion of the pelvis in the hip joints is noticeable because the low back remains in a flexed position.

Panel d. Sitting on the Swiss ball improves the forward head posture only slightly because the lack of mobility and shortness of muscles prevents upright posture. Until mobility of the spine, muscles, and soft tissues are restored, the writer would benefit from a larger ball (65 instead of 55 cm diameter). This would accommodate for the lack of active hip flexion and enable the head to be positioned where the gaze to the screen is in a slight downward direction. This figure also

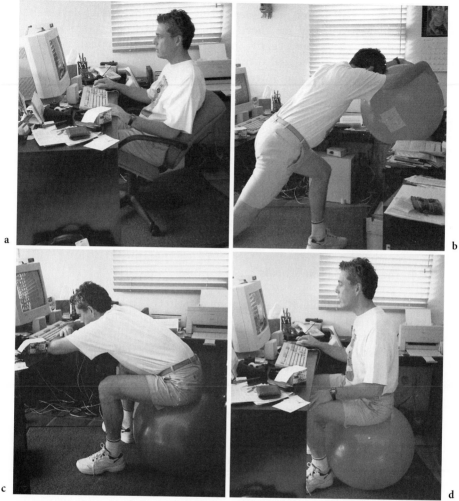

Fig. 15.8 a. A writer who spends most of the day at the computer demonstrates his sitting posture. **b.** Even in a small office the Swiss ball can be used to mobilize the spine into extension while placing the ball on top of the desk. **c.** Rolling the Swiss ball backward while leaning with the forearms on the desk helps to extend the back while flexing the hips. **d.** Sitting on the Swiss ball improves the forward head posture slightly. The writer would benefit from a larger ball because of his decreased active hip flexion.

demonstrates the importance of adjusting the ball to the proportions of the person sitting on it.

> **The Swiss ball is not recommended as a constant seating device. It should be used only for short periods to stretch and mobilize the spine and give proprioceptive input for proper alignment. A good chair should be used for sitting long periods of time. Sitting on a Swiss ball does not guarantee that the patient maintains a good posture unless he has good body awareness.**

The Sitfit (see Chapter 8) or similar sitting devices can help to relieve back strain for some people who sit for long periods at work. Although such a device may make sitting more dynamic, a good chair with a back and arm rests adjusted to the person's proportions is indispensable when working at a desk (Lear and Pomeroy 1994a,b).

It may be very helpful to choose a seat which can be tilted downward independently from the movement of the back support.

15.4.4 The Swiss Ball in Schools

In contrast to the United States, it is not unheard of in Switzerland or Germany to have entire school classes sit on Swiss balls. In Basel, Switzerland, for example, school teachers have been able since 1991 to take courses on how to use the Swiss ball in the classroom (Mühleman et al. 1995). At the beginning of 1995, 14 of 26 elementary school teachers in Basel prescribed that all of their pupils could sit on Swiss balls during class. (In 12 classes 50% of the children or fewer selected Swiss balls instead of chairs. Ten of the children interviewed stated that they preferred conventional chairs for sitting in the class room.)

Most of the teachers had attended an introductory course on the use of the ball in the classrooms, and they monitored the size of the balls and the height of the desks between two and six times per year. This is important in children who are growing rapidly. A survey was conducted among the teachers regarding the effect which the introduction of the Swiss ball had on tension and restlessness: 33% reported a decrease, 25% an increase, and 9% no change (33% did not respond). Asked about the advantages of using the ball in the classroom one teacher answered that the back could move more easily, there was a greater awareness of sitting posture, and there were other possibilities to use the ball. Other teachers reported that emotions of the students became more transparent when sitting on the ball. *Amazingly there were fewer falls from the balls than from chairs.*

The disadvantages that were reported included the balls losing air and being easily damaged, greater space requirements, hygiene, and the noise of the ball.

There has been criticism in German newspapers of the use of Swiss balls instead of chairs (e.g., Anonymous 1996) in regard to both schools and offices. The principal objection is that it is not always practical to sit on a ball (e.g., it is much more difficult to move from the personal computer to other desk equipment while sitting on the ball rather than in a chair with wheels). In chairs without back support many persons tend to slouch, even when sitting on the ball. It is therefore recommended to sit on an ergonomically fitted chair and switch for shorter periods to a Swiss ball.

> Just as it is recommended for other healthy persons, it may be beneficial for some children to sit at times on the Swiss ball. Many classes could benefit from having several Swiss balls to be used as an alternative temporary sitting device.

The Swiss ball remains a great tool for exercising healthy children and adults if they are properly instructed and the balls are indeed used primarily as such.

15.4.5 Relief of Aches and Pains in Health Professionals

Physical therapists familiar with the Swiss ball can attest to the benefit that it can provide after a workday in the hospital that has involved lifting and working with heavy and paralyzed patients. Stretching, moving the back in all planes and in total flexion or extension, and using the ball as a support when working with patients reduces the physical therapist's stress and can alleviate pain and fatigue in the back.

> Whenever the Swiss ball is used, common sense and good judgment is advised. Good observation and listening skills can help the therapist analyze and understand its applications and benefits. The Swiss ball can help the user to maintain or restore mobility, strength, balance, coordination, and skill. Swiss ball exercises should never cause pain.

References

Anderson R (1992) The back pain of bus drivers. Spine 17(12):1481–1487

Anonymous (1996) Eigentor mit dem Sitzball. Westfälische Nachrichten. 27 September

Bejjani FJ, Kaye GM, Benham M (1996) Musculoskeletal and neuromuscular conditions of instrumental musicians. Arch Phys Med Rehabil 77:406–413

Blum J (1995) Der Musiker als physiotherapeutischer Patient – Prävention und Rehabilitation. Krankengymnastik 47(10):1391–1408

Bold RM, Grossmann A (1989) Stemmführung nach R. Brunkow, 5th edn. Enke, Stuttgart

Bork BE, Cook TM, Rosecrance JC, Engelhardt KA, Thomason MEJ, Wauford II, Worley RK (1996) Work-related musculoskeletal disorders among physical therapists. Phys Ther 76(8):827–835

Broich I (1996) Aspekte der Bewegungsentwicklung und des Bewegungsverhalten in der Kieferorthopädie. Krankengymnastik 48(10):1512–1530

Byl NN, Arriaga R (1993) Treating the injured musician. PT Magazine Phys Ther 10:62–68

Fry HJ (1986) Incidence of overuse syndrome in the symphony orchestra. Med Probl Performing Artists 1:51–55

Janda V (1991) Muscle spasm – a proposed procedure for differential diagnosis. Manual Med 6:136–139

Janda V (1994) Manuelle Muskelfunktionsdiagnostik, 3rd edn. Ullstein Mosby, Berlin

Kendall FP, McCreary EK, Provance PG (1993) Muscles: testing and function, 4th edn. Williams & Wilkins, Baltimore

Klein-Vogelbach S (1990) Functional kinetics. Springer, Berlin Heidelberg New York

Klein-Vogelbach S (1991) Therapeutic exercises in functional kinetics. Springer, Berlin Heidelberg New York

Lear CA, Pomeroy SJ (1994a) Office ergonomics. I. The anatomy of seated work. PT Forum 13(24):3–5

Lear CA, Pomeroy SJ (1994b) Office ergonomics. II. General considerations. PT Forum (14)25:3–4

Lederman RJ (1987) Thoracic outlet syndromes. Review of the controversies and a report of 17 instrumental musicians. Med Probl Performing Artists 2:87–91

Mühlemann R, Rühl W, Feierabend A, Amstad H (1995) Basler Primarklassen auf dem Sitzball – eine Bestandesaufnahme 1990–1995. Basler Schulblatt, pp 8–10

Nelson SH (1989) Playing with the entire self: the Feldenkrais method and musicians. Semin Neurol 9(2):97–104

Posner-Mayer, J, Zappala L (1993) FitBall. Ball Dynamics International, Denver

Rosenthal E (1987) The Alexander technique – what it is and how it works. Med Probl Performing Artists 2:52–57

Sahrman SA (1993) Movement as a cause of musculoskeletal pain. In: Singer KP (ed) Integrating approach. Proceedings of the Eighth Biennial Conference of the Manipulative Physical Therapists Association of Australia, pp 69–74

Sandin KJ (1989) The neuromusculoskeletal problems of instrumental musicians: a review. Curr Concepts Rehabil Med 5(1):22–29

Subject Index

An "*f*" following the page numbers indicates figures are included.